Smoking
for Two

Smoking for Two

Cigarettes and Pregnancy

Peter A. Fried
Harry Oxorn

THE FREE PRESS
A Division of Macmillan Publishing Co., Inc.
NEW YORK

Collier Macmillan Publishers
LONDON

The Free Press
A Division of Macmillan Publishing Co., Inc.
866 Third Avenue, New York, N. Y. 10022

Collier Macmillan Canada, Ltd.

Library of Congress Catalog Card Number: 80-20054

Printed in the United States of America

printing number
1 2 3 4 5 6 7 8 9 10

Library of Congress Cataloging in Publication Data

Fred, Peter A
   Smoking for two.

   Bibliography: p.
   Includes index.
      1. Tobacco—Physiological effect. 2. Tobacco—
   Toxicology. 3. Fetus—Effect of drugs on.
   4. Pregnant women—Tobacco use. 5. Pregnancy, Compli-
   cations of. I. Oxorn, Harry, joint author. II. Ti-
   tle.
   RG627.6.T6F74   618.3'2   80-20054
   ISBN 0-02-910720-2

More than most,
this book clearly must be dedicated
to our mothers.

Contents

Contents

Preface

This book has been written in response to a need. The expectant mother is fully aware that with the arrival of her baby her life is going to be altered in a major fashion. It is only natural and right that the pregnant woman's thoughts be dominated by the unborn child, its passage through pregnancy, the birth, and the development of the newborn baby.

From anonymous questionnaires given to mothers-to-be it has been estimated that more than three out of four expectant women read books about pregnancy. They certainly have a wide choice. A trip to a library or bookstore shows quite plainly the wide recognition that the mother-to-be wants to understand what is going on during all stages of her pregnancy. Between 1970 and 1978 over one hundred fifty books were published on topics related to pregnancy. The areas covered are numerous and diverse, including the physiological aspects of pregnancy, caring for the unborn child, childbirth, nutritional considerations for the mother, birth defects, nursing, and coping with the expectant father.

The adages warning that a little knowledge is a dangerous thing and that ignorance is bliss are not accepted by pregnant women. Rightly so! Expectant mothers recognize that they are much more than passive carriers of the unborn. Women have the option of taking an active and informed role during pregnancy. Perhaps the most recent example of this trend is the tremendous interest in Frederick Leboyer's *Birth without Violence*, a book that has led many mothers to discuss with their doctors alternative ways in which babies may be brought into the world.

One realm in which the expectant mother should play an ac-

tive part is in the interaction between the developing fetus and outside influences. Since the Thalidomide tragedy of the early 1960s
pregnant women have been very conscious of the effects drugs
might have. Drugs that may be harmless for the mother are no
longer assumed to be safe for the unborn child. Furthermore, drugs
that may have a particular effect on the pregnant woman are now
recognized as having the potential for quite different and unex-
pected effects on the developing fetus. It is not only the nature of
the drug that determines its effect upon the unborn but also,
because various organs develop at different stages throughout the
pregnancy, the timing of the unborn child's exposure to the substance is of critical significance.

During the course of a pregnancy women are exposed to a
wide variety of drugs, including prescribed medicines, nutritional
supplements, over-the-counter remedies, and socially used substances. Of all of these categories it is the last over which women
can exert the most control by making the decision to take or not to
take them. By socially used drugs we are referring to such substances as nicotine in cigarettes, alcohol, and marijuana. Generally, the social consumption of alcohol (as distinct from alcohol-
ism) and the social use of marijuana aim specifically to make the
user have a sense of well-being. There is not a feeling of compulsion behind their use. Thus, to eschew these substances is relatively
easy. However, for the regular smoker this is not the case.

Smoking is a form of addiction and although the cessation of
smoking is notoriously difficult it can, of course, be accomplished.
The difference in the degree of difficulty in giving up smoking compared to that in giving up regular heavy social drinking (a drink or
two four or five nights a week) is demonstrated vividly in a study
presently under way. In this investigation questionnaires are given
to women who are in various stages of pregnancy. Among other
things inquiries are made about smoking and drinking habits prior
to and during pregnancy. Once pregnancy had been confirmed,
the number of women who became abstainers or extremely light
drinkers more than doubled compared to prepregnancy rates but
the smoking habits of the women remained virtually unchanged.

Two general sets of factors are instrumental in determining
whether a mother-to-be who smokes will stop or not. On one side
are the various physical discomforts, mental anxieties, and changes

in eating habits that accompany the stopping of a longtime cigarette habit. Counterbalancing these potentially substantial discomforts is the fear of the influence of nicotine upon the unborn fetus and, in some cases, a developing aversion to the smoking habit.

But what are the effects of smoking during pregnancy? Surprisingly, there is no in-depth treatment of this question available for the mother-to-be. Many books dealing with the care of the unborn child touch on the subject but rarely are more than two or three pages devoted to this very complex and important issue. We hope that this book will fill the void. By presenting the facts that are known and also by indicating what is not known we will provide expectant mothers (and other interested and concerned individuals) with the information that is needed in order to make a decision about smoking during pregnancy.

To how many individuals is this issue of cigarette smoking and pregnancy relevant? In 1976 American and Canadian governmental statistics indicated that over three and a half million North American women gave birth. Statistics also reveal that about one-third of women of reproductive age smoke on a regular basis. Using these figures we can calculate that over a million women who delivered in 1976 probably smoked during pregnancy. Although that figure is large, the issue of smoking and pregnancy is of concern to a wider population than just expectant mothers who smoke. Without a doubt the father of the unborn child, relatives, and friends would also consider information on smoking and pregnancy as being of considerable importance.

In addition to the smoking mother-to-be and the people who interact with her, there is another group of individuals who also ought to be well informed about the effects of smoking on the unborn. We are talking about the mother-to-be who is a so-called involuntary, or passive smoker. These women do not use cigarettes themselves but through close contact with people who do smoke are forced to inhale the products of smoking. Situations in which regular involuntary inhalation can occur are numerous—the home if the husband smokes, the office, car pools, and other enclosed areas that are frequented by the mother-to-be. Obviously, the number of expectant women who are exposed to these situations cannot be specified but certainly the figure is large.

Preface

This book has been written for all these concerned individuals. All too often much of the information available on smoking and pregnancy is communicated by television, radio, magazines, and newspapers. By their very nature these media emphasize items that can make news headlines, and all too frequently content is condensed to such a degree that considerable distortion of the facts results. Certainly much of the blame for this state of affairs must rest on the shoulders of researchers and physicians. There has been a notorious failure of scientists to communicate their findings directly to the people who are most concerned—the general public.

This situation is gradually changing. We hope that the information presented in this book will serve as a further step in diminishing that communication gap. The pregnant woman or the woman planning to have a baby is particularly receptive to objective information as she considers decisions that may involve changing lifelong habits. This receptiveness comes in large part from the realization that these habits can affect not only her own well-being but also the well-being of her unborn child.

As this book is written for a general audience we have not identified various sources and authorities in the text. This information is available to the reader, however, in the suggested reading list at the end of the book. Nevertheless, it must be emphasized that a large number of studies, many heroic in size and concept, served as the basis for this volume and our indebtedness to many researchers is gratefully acknowledged.

Our appreciation must also be extended to the individuals who helped in different ways at various times in the writing and preparation of this book. These include Rusty Wendt, Jackie Scott, Andrea Grant, Marg Buckingham, Barb Watkinson, Susan Warchow, and Sandy Rochon. The practical, critical, and, most important, moral support of Elfie Fried deserves a special thanks. Finally, but far from least, the inspiration and the raison d'être for the chapters that follow—the many, many mothers-to-be with whom we have had the privilege of sharing, in a sense, their future family addition.

Introduction

A well-known university professor used to start his first class every fall with a dire warning: "Each of you sitting out there in the classroom turn and take a good look at your neighbors on your right and left. By the time the Christmas exams are finished only two of the three of you will still be here." Whether or not this prophesy was fulfilled did not really matter, the not so subtle point of the likelihood of not making it was made quite effectively. Let us use a similar sort of approach to highlight something completely different. If you are a woman between the ages of eighteen and thirty-five, the next time you are in a gathering of women of your own age group consider the women to the right and left. Does one of the three of you smoke? Is one of you planning to have children in the next few years? Chances are the answer to both of these questions is yes. By putting these two things together it is not difficult to see that a considerable percentage of women who are presently pregnant or who are planning to become pregnant probably smoke cigarettes. What is the relationship between smoking and pregnancy? This is a surprisingly complex issue with some aspects still far from resolved.

During the summer of 1978, several psychologists at Carleton University in Ottawa started a long-term investigation of soft drug use during pregnancy. Included in the list of soft drugs were cigarettes. The purpose of the study was twofold. The first objective was to establish an accurate picture of the number of mothers-to-be who used soft drugs either before or during pregnancy and those who did not. The second aim of the study was to examine the effects of these drugs upon the offspring both at birth and after a few months. In order for such a project to get off the ground, a host of factors had to mesh much like gears in a complex machine. Among the cogs that had to roll into action were submissions to governmental and private agencies for funding, the cooperation and support of obstetricians and hospitals, detailed consideration by ethics committees at both the university and the hospitals, and, most essential of all, the interest of mothers-to-be. It was the last aspect that served as the impetus for writing this book.

The format that was followed in the study was that women, upon visiting the gynecologist, were given a short letter by the doctor or nurse that described the purpose of the project. In the letter and in the discussions between patients and doctors that followed, it was emphasized that all pregnant women, whether they smoked, drank, or did neither, were of equal interest, as conclusions could be drawn only by comparing users with nonusers. If the mother-to-be was interested in participating or in obtaining further information an interview was arranged, usually at the home of the woman. At this interview the project was explained in depth and the mother-to-be decided whether or not she wished to participate. If she chose to participate, a detailed questionnaire was given. During this time and usually over a cup of coffee afterward (and occasionally even a cigarette) a discussion took place that centered on the effects of cigarettes on the baby. The women had a chance to ask questions and *all* of them asked about the connection between smoking and pregnancy related topics. Some areas of concern were broad. For example, "Does smoking really affect the baby?" Others were specific: "What happens to the breast milk if I smoke only during the first three months of pregnancy?" Perphaps the most frequently asked question concerned the relation-

2

ship between smoking and the size of the newborn. Very often this question would be phrased "I know that smoking during pregnancy is supposed to cause smaller babies but my sister [or neighbor, or cousin, etc.] smokes like a chimney and her baby was over eight pounds. Why?"

The answers to these and many other questions involved fascinating discussions that invariably included a description of how the fetus develops and the interaction between the fetus and the mother. Very often the conversation would end with the mother-to-be asking where she could get further information on the effects of smoking on pregnancy in a language she could understand. Here we were stuck. The information that we were using in answering the questions came from a variety of sources—medical books, government bulletins, psychological and sociological journals, and other such professional publications. Not only are these items difficult to obtain but they are very often written with specialists in mind.

It was this interest of "our" mothers that prompted the writing of this book. In it we have attempted to describe clearly what is known and what is not known about smoking and pregnancy and to do so in such a manner that the reader does not require any special background. The information contained in the following pages has not been selected to present one side or another of the debate on smoking and pregnancy. Rather, the facts that will be described are just that: facts. This highly complex issue is broken down into a number of subtopics, each with its own chapter. Furthermore, in order to provide not only a description of the effects of smoking but also an explanation of how the effects may (or may not) come about, many of the chapters include a description of the way the body acts and reacts, the mechanisms that underlie such things as fetal growth, the functioning of the placenta, and the manner in which mother and fetus interact.

The topics we discuss include the various questions

asked by the mothers-to-be during interviews, as well as issues that came up in discussions with doctors and scientists doing research in the area of pregnancy and smoking. In Chapter 1 a picture is painted of the extent of smoking among men and women in general, women of all ages, and women of reproductive age. The procedures of obtaining such information are also discussed. Following the description of women who actively smoke we deal in Chapter 2 with another type of smoker—the so-called involuntary smoker—a nonsmoker who frequently finds herself in close quarters with smokers and thus is forced to inhale their smoke. Although relatively little research has been done in this area it certainly is an important concern of many women. After these discussions of both voluntary and involuntary smokers, we move on to specific issues in pregnancy, covering them in a more or less logical time sequence. A description of some of the possible mechanisms by which cigarette smoke may affect the pregnant woman and her unborn child is provided in Chapter 3. With this background we deal in Chapter 4 with maternal weight gain, what it reflects, and how smoking may affect it. From there, in Chapter 5, we deal with the amazing system of communication between the mother and fetus—the placenta. This organ serves in part as a selective filter between the mother's system and the baby's system and therefore determines to a considerable extent the degree to which the contents of cigarette smoke will affect the fetus. Chapter 6 considers the possible link between smoking and complications during pregnancy. Chapter 7 discusses full term and premature babies, how a baby is defined as premature, the data relating smoking to the length of gestation, and the interaction of cigarettes and the birth weight of the infant. An astounding number of newborns have been evaluated with respect to the last issue. In many hospitals the newborn is tested and examined at birth for a host of factors including general health, activity, functioning of the nervous system, and the working of the respiratory and cardiovascular systems. We will discuss some of these tests in Chapter 8 and whether or not smoking during pregnancy affects the results. Of course, during pregnancy not only is the fetus continuously undergoing dramatic changes but also the mother in many ways is biologically being prepared for the birth and events immediately afterward. One of the preparations consists of readying the mother for nursing the baby. Therefore, the production of milk, its nutritional value, and the effects of smoking upon the milk produced are dealt with in Chapter 9. In Chapter 10 the studies that have examined the possible long-term effects of smoking during pregnancy are discussed. That is, is there any evidence that smoking during fetal development can influence a youngster of three or four? How would such effects manifest themselves? Finally, in Chapter 11 we deal with the consequences of stopping a longtime smoking habit. Throughout the various chapters we will be emphasizing where information is relatively complete and where, on the other hand, the relationship between smoking and a particular phenomenon is either tentative or merely speculative.

Perhaps at the very outset, before proceeding to the information derived from a large number of studies, a clear statement should be made concerning how results ought to be interpreted. Earlier we mentioned the mother-to-be who wondered whether smoking during pregnancy is associated with lower birth weight. She was skeptical because someone she knew who was a heavy smoker had given birth to a large baby. At issue here is something called probability, or likelihood. When you go to a horse race and place a bet, what you are actually doing is guessing the likelihood of your horse's winning. A similar sort of thing occurs when one interprets the results of a scientific study—although it is hoped that more than guessing is involved. For example, the studies that report a relationship between smoking and birth weight express the results in terms of probabilities. That is, if you were a gambler or a betting person, the results of the studies would give you a fair idea what the odds would be of a heavy smoker's having a smaller baby than a mother who was a nonsmoker but similar in other respects. But, as in virtually all other betting situations, even if the likelihood (or odds) is known, the outcome is not a sure thing. There will always be exceptions that go against the odds. How often such exceptions occur depends upon how great the likelihood is that smoking is related to reduced birth weight. The greater the probability that smoking and smaller babies are related, the fewer the exceptions to the rule.

Whether one is talking about gambling at the racetrack or the results from a scientific study, probabilities have values that range from zero to one. If we are certain that a particular event or relationship will never occur, then the probability is described as zero. On the other hand, if we know for certain that a particular event will always occur, the probability can be stated as one (or 100 percent). In this book it will be extremely rare to find any relationship that can be expressed in terms of 100 percent probability, or, in other words, absolute certainty.

The factors discussed in the following chapters will have probability values that lie between zero and one. This means that over the long run a particular event is expected to occur a certain percentage of the time. For example, if the relationship between smoking and a particular effect in the newborn has a probability of 0.85, that effect would be expected to occur 85 percent of the time in a long series of observations of newborns born to smoking mothers. In this example, the probability lets us make an educated guess as to what is going to happen when a smoking mother gives birth. We would call this the risk factor for this particular effect, a risk factor of 0.85. But, because the probability is neither zero nor one we cannot be certain. We can only go with the odds. Of course, by knowing the probability we are more likely to be right than is the person who attempts to predict what is going to happen without knowing the odds.

Sometimes the probability assigned to a particular event or relationship is determined by analyzing the physical characteristics of the device or situation that is producing the event. The fact that a coin is evenly balanced and has only two sides, a heads and a tails, enables us to predict that the likelihood of throwing a tails is one chance in two, or a probability of 0.5. In other cases, however, such as our example of horse racing and, more to the point, smoking and pregnancy, the nature of the physical mechanisms are neither completely nor even well understood. Therefore, the probability of events in these circumstances must be determined, at least in part, by observations of the relative frequency in the past of the particular event.

So, when we say that a relationship has been found between smoking and a particular effect upon the fetus, bear in mind that such findings are really expressing a likelihood, or probability, and not a certainty that the effect will occur again in the future.

chapter one
Who Are the Smokers?

The concept of a billion of anything is hard to grasp. One way in which the enormous number can start to be imagined is to relate it to something that is familiar. For example, the atomic bomb was dropped in World War II one billion seconds ago. The Christian era began one billion minutes ago. Men were living in caves one billion hours ago. These figures give one something to think about. But how about the following fact—it is even more staggering: one billion cigarettes were smoked by North Americans between 1978 and 1980.

Almost immediately after the introduction of tobacco into Europe in the sixteenth century there was a recognition of its potential ill effects and campaigns against it were begun. However, neither moral, nor economic, nor health considerations managed to discourage its use. The cigarette came into being during the nineteenth century followed by the necessary machinery for its mass production. By the middle of the present century the use of tobacco was socially completely acceptable among males. The smoking of cigarettes was not considered by most to be a form of drug use. This attitude still exists today to a large degree and the legal status of cigarettes in most countries reflects this view. So, in the United States and Canada controls that are applied to most drugs are not applied to tobacco. It is considered a crop and is treated as an agricultural product.

In the past ten years or so there have been widespread governmental programs informing people of the health hazards associated with smoking. In the same time period there has been a fairly radical shift in the attitudes that society holds toward women, and advertisers have been quick to take full advantage of this development. "You've come a long way, baby" and similarly unsubtle attempts to equate woman's liberation and maturity with smoking in a real sense compete with the health campaigns waged by doctors and governments. Overall, during the 1970s, as the statistics in this chapter will show, if you had to pick a winner in the battle for the minds of young women, the decision would have to go to the advertisers.

In spite of the enormous number of cigarettes smoked during the years 1965–1980 in such countries as the United States, Canada, Great Britain, Sweden, and Australia studies have revealed that there is a general decline in smoking. In the United States, for example, the percentage of regular smokers declined over the ten years from 1965 to 1974 from 53 percent to 39 percent. In Canada during the same period a similar decrease was observed, with the percentage of smokers falling from 45 to 40 percent. The downward shift in the percentage of regular cigarette smokers has been noted to be quite consistent in young and middle-aged males but the trends are not clear among females. This situation can best be seen in Figures 1–1 and 1–2, which describe the proportion of adult smokers in the United States and Canada. The numbers used for the American statistics were obtained by interviews, usually over the phone, with approximately twelve thousand individuals. The figures from Canada were gathered from some seventy-five thousand people in approximately thirty thousand households by means of a written questionnaire.

From the two figures several facts deserve to be noted. Because the data were put together differently in the two countries, the ages of the individuals for which information is available differ slightly. The American data distinguish between twenty-five to thirty-four year olds and thirty-five

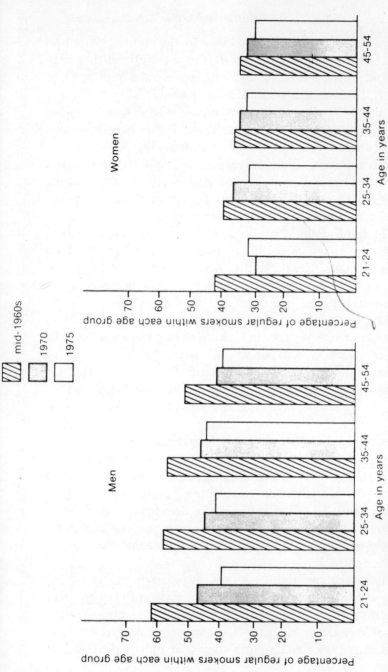

Figure 1-1. Percentage of regular smokers by age group and sex in the United States for the mid-1960s, 1970, and 1975.

10

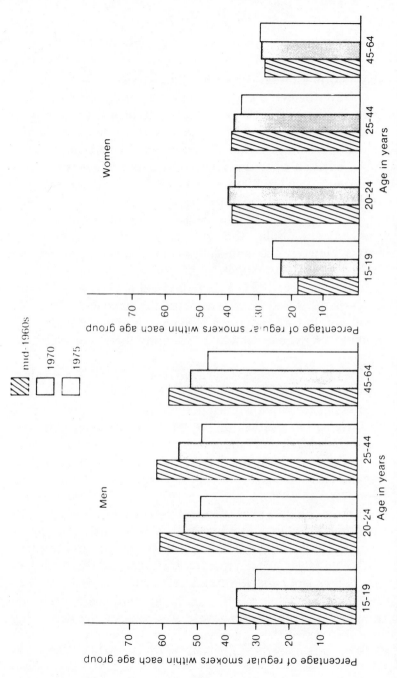

Figure 1–2. Percentage of regular smokers by age group and sex in Canada for the mid-1960s, 1970, and 1975.

11

to forty-four year olds while the Canadian data group these ages together. On the other hand, the Canadian statistics give information on fifteen to nineteen year olds.

Nevertheless, the trends are very similar in both countries. In the mid-1960s the percentage of adult males who smoked was considerably greater than it was in the early and mid-1970s. Thus, in the United States 54 percent of adult males smoked cigarettes regularly in 1965 whereas the percentage dropped to 40 percent in 1975. For Canada the percentage of regular smokers dropped from 58 percent in 1965 to 46 percent in 1975. The data collected for women, however, do not display the same regular decline in smoking habits between the mid-sixties and mid-seventies. In the United States approximately 32 percent of women smoked regularly in 1964. This figure dropped slightly—to 30 percent—in 1970 and remained essentially unchanged in 1975. Similarly, in Canada only a 1 percent drop was noted in the number of women smoking regularly between 1965 and 1975.

Of particular interest are women of the peak reproductive years, approximately eighteen to twenty-eight. The figures illustrate that women in the United States and Canada in their early twenties, unlike their male counterparts, did not change their smoking habits between 1970 and 1975. In fact, Figure 1–2 shows that in Canada the percentage of regular smokers aged fifteen to nineteen gradually increased from 1965 to 1975.

From the data accumulated by the governments of both the United States and Canada it is clear that patterns of smoking over the years have differed for men and women. Although fewer women than men smoke, and those who do are lighter smokers, the trend in North America and elsewhere is that, while men are giving up smoking in increasing numbers, the proportion of women smokers is not decreasing and, in fact, at the younger age level is actually increasing. Putting this point in a nutshell, approximately one-third of

North American women of childbearing age are cigarette smokers.

What has been discussed so far are the smoking habits of women in general and women of reproductive age in particular. But what about women who are pregnant? What are their smoking habits? As one may well imagine it is harder to get information about the smoking habits of mothers-to-be than it is to get similar data from women in the general population. After all, in the latter case just about every second person is a female and thus it is relatively easy to find a large group to question. This is not the case with pregnant women. Nevertheless, several studies have been undertaken in order to answer this important question.

One of the largest studies was carried out in 1960–1961 in ten teaching hospitals in the province of Ontario, Canada. Information was obtained from interviews with over fifty thousand women while they were still in the hospital after having given birth. Approximately 13 percent of the mothers reported that they had smoked a pack or more a day during pregnancy; 30 percent had smoked less than a pack a day; and approximately 50 percent were nonsmokers. By combining these figures it can be seen that approximately 43 percent of the mothers were regular smokers during pregnancy. In this large study the relationship between the age of the mother-to-be and her smoking habit was considered. The researchers, after interviewing the women, divided them up into various age brackets. They found that the younger the mother, the greater was the likelihood that she would be a light smoker, consuming less than a pack a day, as opposed to her being a nonsmoker. However, there was no trend between the age of the mother and those who smoked more than a pack a day. That is, the likelihood of a woman's being a heavy smoker did not differ between the younger and the older mothers.

The fact that slightly over 40 percent of the women in this study reported that they smoked regularly during pregnancy deserves comment. From Figures 1-1 and 1-2 it can be seen that around 1965, approximately 42 percent of women of peak reproductive age reported that they smoked regularly. Most of these women presumably were not pregnant. Looking at the proportion of women who stated that they smoked regularly during pregnancy, the number is also around the 42 percent point. This would suggest that few women in the mid-1960s altered their smoking habits when they became pregnant.

Some data, however, suggest that a number of mothers did alter their smoking habits upon becoming pregnant and smoked less throughout the whole pregnancy. For example, out of 3700 women interviewed in an American hospital in the early 1970s, 50 percent reported smoking in the year preceding their pregnancy. Of these women, approximately a quarter cut down on smoking during the first trimester.

The two most common reasons given by the mothers for this reduction was a feeling of sickness or nausea when they smoked and concern for the infant. The fact that these interviews took place in the hospital shortly after the babies were born may have had some bearing on the responses given. For example, some mothers might have suspected that doctors have a negative attitude toward smoking during pregnancy. Thus, in the hospital they might have tended to give a lower estimate of their smoking habit as compared to the answer they might have given at home to interviewers not perceived as having any particular point of view.

In addition to these North American studies, other large investigations have been undertaken in Europe. For example, in Cardiff, Wales, between 1965 and 1968 approximately eighteen thousand women were interviewed within a few days of having given birth. They were asked about their smoking habits before and during pregnancy. The results were quite similar to those of the Ontario study described earlier in this chapter. In that study, 43 percent of the fifty thousand women interviewed reported that they had smoked during pregnancy. In the Welsh study, carried out approximately six years later, 40 percent of the new mothers reported that they had smoked while pregnant. Not only were the percentages of smokers similar in these two studies but also the number of women who changed their habits once they became pregnant did not differ markedly. In both cases the percentages were quite small. In the Ontario study it was estimated that approximately 1 percent of the women stopped smoking during pregnancy, while in the Welsh study the number was less than 6 percent.

In a Canadian study that is still under way (referred to in the introduction) we have interviewed approximately three hundred women. However, the procedures followed in our investigation differ considerably from the methods used in the other studies described earlier. In the latter, women were interviewed after the birth of the baby. In our work, women are contacted early in pregnancy, typically during the first trimester, and are interviewed several times prior to the birth. Although such a procedure is quite time-consuming it has several advantages. For instance, mothers-to-be have a much better memory for things that happened before they became pregnant if you ask about these things when the woman is still pregnant as opposed to nine months later. Furthermore, by interviewing the mothers-to-be several times during the pregnancy, a more reliable estimate of their smoking habits can be obtained. Finally, because the same interviewer is used for all the question-and-answer sessions, a friendly, informal atmosphere can be established, thus increasing the likelihood of accurate estimates of smoking habits from the pregnant women.

The figures obtained in this study have been somewhat lower than those found in studies in which women were interviewed soon after the birth of the baby. In our study the proportion of women who smoked regularly during the year preceding the pregnancy is approximately one-third.

This is 6 percent less than the percentages found in the

studies based on interviews with women in the early and mid-1960s. As pictured in Figure 1-2, the general rate of smoking in Canadian women (both pregnant and not pregnant) during the peak reproductive years was unchanged from the mid-sixties to the mid-seventies at about 39 percent. In our study the lower figure of 33 percent of women who reported smoking regularly in the year before their pregnancy may represent a downward swing in the percentage of young women smoking. In view of the intensive Canadian government antismoking campaign in the years immediately preceding this study, the decrease in the percentage of regular smokers is not surprising.

When we asked mothers-to-be about their smoking habits before becoming pregnant and during the first trimester, less than 8 percent replied that they had stopped smoking. Later in pregnancy the percentage of women who smoked actually increased slightly as a few women took up the habit once more in the second or third trimester.

The finding in our study that only a small number of women altered their smoking habits is consistent with that of a 1971 Swedish investigation that used a somewhat similar procedure, namely, women were given questionnaires each time they visited their doctor during pregnancy. Their smoking habits before and during pregnancy were determined. As in the North American studies done in the same period—the mid-sixties—just under 45 percent of women smoked before they became pregnant. What is striking is that fewer than one woman in a hundred in the Swedish study stopped smoking after finding out that she was pregnant. In fact, there were almost as many women who started smoking during pregnancy. So, it would seem that although the percentage of women who smoked during the 1960s was considerably greater than that in the late 1970s, the tendency to change smoking habits once a baby is on the way was as negligible as it appears to be today.

In our ongoing project an additional interesting finding

has turned up in asking the mothers-to-be about their husbands' smoking habits. About 40 percent of the women reported that their husbands smoked during the pregnancy. This figure is approximately 7 percent less than that found in 1975 among males of a similar age. It would appear that the downward trend in women smokers of childbearing age described earlier is also present in men of comparable age. The percentage shift is virtually the same in both sexes.

What about the number of households in which both males and females smoke? Or, conversely, in how many cases does one person smoke but the other not? In our study we have found that over half of the husbands who smoked had wives who did not smoke. Conversely, approximately one out of three women who smoked during pregnancy had husbands who did not smoke. Overall during pregnancy, of the women who smoked, just over half did so in a household where the husband also smoked. These figures reveal no clear pattern of smoking within families. It is not possible given that either the husband or the wife smokes to predict the smoking habits of the spouse. Of particular interest for our purpose is the case in which the mother-to-be does not smoke but lives in a house in which she is repeatedly exposed to the exhaled smoke of someone else's cigarette. This situation will be discussed in detail in the next chapter.

What can we say after seeing all these figures? Certainly, a large number of women who are pregnant or who may be contemplating getting pregnant do smoke. Furthermore, only a small percentage of women change their smoking habits once they find out that they are to be a mother. And, finally, even if the woman does not smoke during pregnancy, she may nonetheless be exposed to cigarette smoke on a regular basis.

chapter two

Involuntary Smokers

In the previous chapter it was pointed out that a considerable percentage of pregnant women who are nonsmokers are married to men who smoke. Thus, it is reasonable to presume that in these cases the mother-to-be frequently has to breathe air that contains a considerable amount of cigarette smoke. Of course, this exposure to someone else's smoke is not restricted to the home. The workplace is another likely location in which nonsmokers may regularly be exposed to tobacco smoke. In countless other situations, too, such as in cars or trains and at sporting events and parties, the nonsmoker, by the very act of breathing, is exposed to many of the constituents of tobacco smoke that are inhaled by the person actually holding the cigarette to his or her lips. For obvious reasons this sort of exposure is called passive smoking, or involuntary smoking. It is passive in that the nonsmoker is not actively doing anything except the very natural (and necessary) act of breathing; it is involuntary because the smoke is inhaled as an unavoidable result of breathing.

The smoke contained in the air in situations like this actually comes from two sources. There is the smoke that is exhaled by smokers after they have drawn it through the cigarette. This is usually referred to as mainstream smoke. There is also sidestream smoke, or smoke that leaves the burning tip of the cigarette between puffs.

Mainstream and sidestream smoke put different things into the air. There are a number of reasons for this difference. In part it has to do with what happens to smoke inside the lungs of the active smoker. For example, when the smoker inhales, his or her lungs absorb a considerable amount of carbon monoxide and nicotine. As a result, the exhaled smoke contains considerably less of these substances than does sidestream smoke. So if you are a passive smoker, the content of the air you are inhaling will depend to a considerable degree upon the depth of inhalation by the active smoker. A host of other factors also come into play when evaluating the smoke to which an involuntary smoker is exposed. For instance, how much ventilation is available for the removal of smoke? How close is the nonsmoker to the smoker? How long and how regularly is the passive smoker exposed to cigarette smoke? Keep in mind that when the smoker inhales and exhales he or she does so about nine times per cigarette, making the actual smoking time only about twenty-four seconds. But the cigarette produces smoke for about twenty-five times that length of time and therefore the passive smoker is exposed to sidestream smoke for about twelve minutes.

What is known about the effects of involuntary inhalation? Although a number of studies have examined this question using individuals of varying ages and varying degrees of health, no investigation has specifically studied the involuntary pregnant smoker. In spite of this unfortunate absence, it is worthwhile to look at the findings obtained from nonpregnant individuals and to see whether they can at least suggest how passive inhalation may affect a mother-to-be.

You'll recall that substances such as nicotine and carbon monoxide are found in lower concentrations in mainstream (or exhaled) smoke as compared to sidestream smoke. For example there may be up to twice as much nicotine and five times as much carbon monoxide in sidestream smoke compared to mainstream smoke. This means that involuntary smoke inhalation differs in content as well as in amount from active smoke inhalation by a smoker. One of the major products of burning tobacco is carbon monoxide. Various government agencies such as the United States Environmental Protection Agency have determined the maximum acceptable amount of carbon monoxide in the air (in terms of general, more or less continuous exposure) to be nine parts of carbon monoxide per million parts of air.

The level of carbon monoxide present in an enclosed area in which people are smoking is influenced largely by three factors. The size of the area in which the smoking occurs will determine the concentration of carbon monoxide in the air. A second factor is the number and type of tobacco products being smoked. For example, cigars contain more carbon monoxide per puff than do either filtered or unfiltered cigarettes or even pipes. The amount and efficiency of ventilation is the third factor that plays an important role in determining carbon monoxide levels. Furthermore, the carbon monoxide levels are higher if a given number of cigarettes are smoked at one time rather than one after another. So, for example, a greater amount of carbon monoxide would be produced by four cigarettes smoked at the same time than by four cigarettes smoked in a row.

Given that these three factors—the size of the enclosed area, the quantity and types of tobacco product being smoked, and the kind of ventilation—are crucial in determining carbon monoxide levels in the air and keeping in mind that nine parts carbon monoxide per million parts of air is considered the maximum acceptable level for extended periods of time, what are the levels of carbon monoxide in a number of typical situations?

In a moderate-sized car with no ventilation ten cigarettes smoked over the course of an hour were found to produce carbon monoxide levels approximately ten times the acceptable level. Having the vents and blower on in the car, thereby providing ventilation, reduces the carbon monoxide level considerably, although the extent of the reduction obviously depends on the size of the air vents and the efficiency of the blower. In some studies carbon monoxide levels were reduced by one-third, in others by over two-thirds. But in all studies in which four or more cigarettes were smoked, the carbon monoxide level exceeded the maximum acceptable level of nine parts per million.

Studies conducted in various sized rooms have also been undertaken. In an office the approximate size of a large living room, with three employees who smoked, the air was found to have a carbon monoxide level of fifteen parts per million. When the rooms were ventilated by means of open windows or air conditioning, the carbon monoxide levels were usually reported as being below the maximum acceptable concentration.

Knowing the concentration of carbon monoxide in the air is only one of the steps in assessing the effects this substance may have upon the passive smoker. What is also of importance is the amount actually absorbed by the involuntary smoker. Quite obviously, as the concentration of carbon monoxide increases in the air around the nonsmoker, so does the amount inhaled. But other factors also enter into this state of affairs. For example, how rapidly is the passive smoker breathing? If the involuntary smoker is doing hard labor or is exercising, the rate of respiration will be faster and the breaths deeper than if the individual were just sitting quietly.

One method of determining the amount of carbon monoxide actually inhaled by somebody is to analyze a certain constituent of the blood, namely, hemoglobin. Normally, one of the functions of hemoglobin is to carry essential oxygen throughout the body. When carbon monoxide is absorbed it becomes attached to the hemoglobin and prevents the hemoglobin from carrying its normal load of oxygen. The more carbon monoxide that is inhaled, the less hemoglobin available for doing its normal job. Carbon monoxide and hemoglobin combine to form a substance called carboxyhemoglobin. The levels of this compound can be measured

21

and the number obtained serves as an indicator of the amount of carbon monoxide absorbed.

Using this index, it has been found that if the concentration of carbon monoxide in the air is less than the maximum acceptable level, increase in carboxyhemoglobin is minimal. However, when the carbon monoxide level in the air reaches a concentration that is judged to be as great or greater than is present in most social situations (thirty parts carbon monoxide per million parts of air), the level of carboxyhemoglobin in the blood more than doubles within two hours. Even though this is a considerable increase, medical evidence indicates that the actual amount of carboxyhemoglobin formed probably has an insignificant effect on the healthy adult. However, in individuals with heart disease, carbon monoxide inhaled by involuntary smoking may seriously strain the functioning of the heart. This effect occurs even in a well-ventilated room. Blood pressure and heart rate are both increased in passive smokers with certain heart problems following exposure to cigarette smoke, presumably because of increased levels of carboxyhemoglobin. Increased carboxyhemoglobin levels mean less oxygen available to the heart, making it work harder; because of the heart's diseased state, there could be severe consequences.

As we mentioned near the beginning of this chapter, there have been no reports on the effects of passive smoking by pregnant women. But we do know that during pregnancy both the mother-to-be and the developing baby have physiological demands placed upon them that increase the woman's need for oxygen. In a mother-to-be the respiratory rate increases. There are probably two reasons for this result. Space is taken up by the growing fetus that in the nonpregnant woman is normally occupied by the lungs as they fill with air during inhalation. Since the mother-to-be cannot get as much air into her lungs as normal she compensates by breathing more rapidly. But there is an important additional factor that requires the mother-to-be to breathe at a rate that is even faster than the reduced capacity of the lungs would dictate. That factor is the oxygen needs of the growing fetus. Later on in this book we will discuss the needs of the unborn baby. At this time let us say that as the baby is developing among the many demands that he or she places upon the mother is the demand for a considerable amount of oxygen. The baby in the womb cannot get the oxygen he or she needs directly from the air and has to rely on satisfying his or her requirements by using the mother as a transport system. The mother's bloodstream, with its hemoglobin, therefore has to carry enough oxygen obtained from the air in her lungs to satisfy both her needs and the baby's needs. This double requirement is partially met by an increase in the respiratory rate of the mother.

Therefore, what we have in the case of a pregnant woman exposed to the cigarette smoke of others is an individual who is absorbing carbon monoxide at a somewhat greater rate than is a comparable nonpregnant woman in the same environment. Presumably the formation of carboxy-hemoglobin would be higher in the mother-to-be at a time when her oxygen requirements are somewhat higher because of the demands of the fetus.

Much the same sort of story can be told about the heart of the mother-to-be. During pregnancy the number of heartbeats per minute in the mother increases from approximately seventy to around ninety. This rise in the number of contractions of the heart places an extra demand on the heart muscle, thereby increasing its need for oxygen. The heart of the fetus, which starts beating approximately ten weeks after conception, also has a high rate of contraction—about 140 beats per minute—and thus has great oxygen needs. So, during pregnancy the hearts of both the mother-to-be and the developing baby are working at a high rate with correspondingly great oxygen needs.

Thus, although no direct work has been done on the effects of carbon monoxide on the pregnant passive smoker, it seems reasonable to deduce that because respiration rate is increased during pregnancy, inhalation of sidestream and mainstream smoke is therefore greater during pregnancy. Also, the oxygen needs of the mother-to-be are greater. This combination makes it clear that elevated levels of carbon monoxide in the air or of carboxyhemoglobin in the blood of pregnant women will have more marked effects than would similar levels in nonpregnant individuals. Furthermore, because of the needs of the growing fetus, the decrease in oxygen carried by the mother-to-be may be of much greater consequence than a similar decrease in a woman not carrying a developing baby.

Up to this point we have discussed only carbon monoxide inhalation by the passive smoker. The reason for this focus is primarily that more is known about involuntary carbon monoxide inhalation than about inhalation of the other products of smoking. A few studies have examined involuntary inhalation of nicotine. This substance has been linked to cardiovascular disease in cigarette smokers. In the air, nicotine acts quite differently from carbon monoxide. Carbon monoxide tends to remain in the air until it is removed by ventilation or other means. Nicotine, on the other hand, does not linger but settles out of the air on its own. Thus, after smoking has ceased, the amount of nicotine in the air to which the involuntary smoker is exposed diminishes.

As with carbon monoxide no studies have looked at nicotine and the pregnant passive smoker. In nonpregnant involuntary smokers the levels of nicotine absorbed during passive inhalation have been assessed by an analysis of urine. In a smoke-filled room the nicotine level of passive smokers is only 1 percent of that found in active smokers. Very slight increases in nicotine level among involuntary smokers were also found in sailors on board a submarine that was well ventilated but staffed by a large number of smokers.

On the basis of these few studies it seems unlikely that the small amounts of nicotine absorbed by passive smokers, pregnant or not, would be a major factor in terms of health effects.

One final comment about passive smoking refers to the rather common complaint from nonsmokers of minor eye and throat irritations, which are more pronounced in warm, dry air (e.g., a heated home in winter). Although these symptoms do not constitute any direct health hazard to the developing fetus, the probability that prolonged throat irritation may lead to respiratory disease in the mother-to-be should not be overlooked. Along these lines, it is worthwhile to mention that children who live in a household in which one or both of the parents smoke are more likely to have respiratory infections such as bronchitis and pneumonia than are children living in nonsmoking families.

In summary, then, although no direct work has been done on the effects of passive smoking upon the pregnant woman, the implications from other studies are numerous. Exposure to air containing a fair amount of cigarette smoke has, as its principal effect, the reduction of the oxygen-carrying capacity of the mother-to-be. Whether this reduction is severe enough to affect the fetus, even under heavy exposure conditions such as in a car or in a small room, has not been determined. But certainly it can be stated that any diminution in oxygen available to the developing fetus increases the risk to that organism. The degree of that risk remains to be determined and will vary markedly depending upon the various factors discussed earlier in this chapter.

chapter three
Constituents of Smoke

Tobacco smoke is made up of a mixture of gases and tiny droplets of solid matter, mainly tar, in which over a thousand different compounds have been identified. Although some components are filtered off as the smoke is drawn through the unburned tobacco, they are reproduced as the burning ember advances, and the smoke in each successive puff becomes more concentrated. As it enters the mouth, smoke can be thought of as being quite similar to a spray from an aerosal can—with this particular spray containing millions of particles per cubic inch.

Since cigarette smoke is less irritating to the throat than that produced by pipe or cigar smoking, it is more likely to be inhaled. However, while smoking pipes or cigars is less hazardous than smoking cigarettes, it is not completely harmless. For example, regular, noninhaling smokers of pipes and cigars have a higher incidence of cancer of the mouth than do cigarette smokers. Obviously, few pregnant women smoke pipes or cigars and therefore in this book we will be referring almost exclusively to cigarette smokers. However, it should be kept in mind that many a mother-to-be may be exposed to the exhaled and sidestream smoke of pipes and cigars as a passive smoker.

The products of tobacco smoke are absorbed from the mouth, the upper respiratory tract, and the lungs into the bloodstream, in which they are carried to all parts of the body. As we will discuss later, these substances cross the placenta easily and rapidly by a process of simple diffusion and thereby pass from the maternal to the fetal bloodstream.

The most important components of tobacco smoke are nicotine, which acts in the heart, blood vessels, digestive tract, kidneys, and nervous system; carbon monoxide, which, as we have described, interferes with the oxygen-carrying ability of hemoglobin; minute amounts of substances that can produce cancer; and irritants that act on the air passages of the lungs and upper respiratory tract. In spite of the many, many compounds that make up tobacco smoke, only nicotine and carbon monoxide have been studied in any depth with respect to pregnancy and therefore most of our discussion will center around these two.

Nicotine is the most active and most powerful agent in cigarette smoke. In terms of its chemical makeup it is related to a number of drugs known for other properties. For example, nicotine is in the same chemical family as the poison strychnine, the medicine quinine, the hallucinogen mescaline, and the addictive pain relievers cocaine, opium, morphine, heroin, and codeine.

Since the mid-1960s the evidence has been rather convincing that nicotine is a powerful addictive drug and that smoking is a powerful addiction. Although some people do prefer to label smoking an habituating behavior rather than an addiction this distinction appears to be more one of words than facts. Virtually all people working in the area of smoking agree that regular smokers feel a compulsion to have a cigarette in order to experience its effects and sometimes to avoid the discomforts of its absence. What we have here are the two fundamental aspects of an addictive drug: dependence and withdrawal symptoms if the drug is not used.

In fact, today cigarette smoking is probably one of the most dependency producing forms of self-administered gratification known to man and, as we have seen in the first chapter, woman. The potency of the addiction can be seen in the fact that over two-thirds of smokers would like to quit and also have good reasons for wishing to stop yet they are compelled to continue with their habit. Fewer than one in five stop permanently in spite of being aware of the physical harm, expense, and increasing social disapproval associated with smoking. In other words, for most smokers cigarette smoking is a compulsion. An interesting estimate given by a U.S. government official is that over two-thirds of people who ever smoked still smoke on a regular basis. That figure is a powerful argument for considering nicotine a potent addictive drug. This estimate is especially striking when one realizes that less than 15 percent of people who ever used heroin are still addicted to that narcotic.

Other factors associated with addiction are also evident with smoking. Withdrawal symptoms, which occur when a drug upon which a person has become dependent is witheld, are well known to smokers. Often within a few hours after the last cigarette the regular smoker may feel restless, anxious, or depressed and find his or her concentration impaired. Withdrawal signs, as we will discuss in later chapters, may also be evident in babies born to maternal smokers. At birth the baby is suddenly removed from the nicotine, which had been crossing the placenta, and may well suffer physical consequences.

Another phenomenon frequently associated with addictive drugs is tolerance. This condition occurs when a person becomes accustomed to some of the initial effects of a drug. With nicotine tolerance appears to develop. Almost every youngster who smoked his or her first, forbidden cigarette in secret will testify to the initial sensations of dizziness, sweating, and nausea, effects that disappear with regular smoking. Furthermore, if smoking becomes a regular habit, frequently the intake after a year or two will increase as tolerance develops to some of the desired effects of nicotine; that is, more cigarettes will be needed to achieve the same feelings.

The continued use of cigarettes by smokers is related

both to psychological and to pharmacological factors. If one considers that a person who smokes a pack a day actually takes more than fifty thousand nicotine puffs a year, it is not hard to see that one is dealing with a very strong habit that psychologically would be hard to change. Think of anything else done fifty thousand times a year that for some reason must be stopped. Coupled with this difficulty is the fact that pharmacologically nicotine produces effects in the nervous system that also are reinforcing. This phenomenon can be dramatically seen in the failure of nicotine-free tobacco or other plant materials to satisfy the needs of those who have acquired the nicotine habit.

When a puff of cigarette smoke is inhaled, the amount of nicotine absorbed is the equivalent of an injection directly into the vein of 0.1 milligram. Up to two milligrams of nicotine are absorbed from the smoke of a single cigarette. If this amount were injected rather than inhaled rapid death would occur as the centers in the brain controlling the heart and breathing would be paralyzed.

In the amounts absorbed via inhalation during cigarette smoking, nicotine acts on certain specialized bundles of nerves and on the adrenal glands to stimulate a release of chemicals. These chemicals then bring about a variety of effects, including an increase in the heart rate, an increase in the amount of blood pumped by the heart, narrowing of the peripheral blood vessels, a rise in blood pressure, an increase in the concentration of sugar in the blood, and a greater tendency for the blood to clot. The constriction of the blood vessels reduces the amount of blood reaching the tissues. These effects disappear quite quickly after a cigarette is finished.

For a long time it has been recognized that many of the effects seen in smoking adults are also seen in the unborn baby of a mother who smokes. For example, as early as 1935 investigations revealed that there is a definite rise in the fetal heart rate when the mother begins smoking a cigarette and suggested that this effect probably is caused by nicotine passing across the placenta.

The effect of nicotine on the fetus is brought about in two main ways. First, nicotine is a potent constrictor of veins and, by narrowing the maternal blood vessels that supply the uterus, causes a decrease in the amount of blood reaching the placenta and a consequent reduction in the supply of oxygen and food available to the fetus. In addition, nicotine crosses the placenta, enters the fetal circulation, and affects the fetal cardiovascular system. These actions may or may not explain some effects observed among the fetuses of women who smoke. These include lower birth weight, increase in the fetal heart rate, and decrease in the fetal breathing movements while in the uterus. All of these possibilities and their mechanisms will be elaborated in subsequent chapters.

Carbon monoxide is a powerful respiratory poison that can, when present in too great amounts, cause death. Harmful effects may occur even when the concentration in the blood is relatively low.

As we noted in Chapter 3, under normal conditions oxygen in the blood is attached to hemoglobin, an iron-containing constituent of the red blood cells. When normal hemoglobin comes in contact with tissues that require oxygen it gives its oxygen up readily.

Carbon monoxide is absorbed into the lungs from cigarette smoke, reaches the bloodstream, and attaches itself to the hemoglobin to form carboxyhemoglobin. This process has two bad effects. Because carbon monoxide has a two hundred times greater tendency to attach to hemoglobin than does oxygen, it displaces oxygen from the hemoglobin in the red blood cells. This reduces the oxygen-carrying capacity of both the mother and the fetus; there is a reduction in the amount of oxygen carried by each red blood cell. In addition, a high level of carboxyhemoglobin impairs the offloading or transfer of even the reduced amount of oxygen from the hemoglobin to the tissues. Thus, both the oxygen-carrying capacity of the blood and its ability to release oxygen to the tissues are reduced. The most serious effect of carbon monoxide on developing tissue is this interference with the tissues obtaining their essential amount of oxygen.

A small amount of the carbon monoxide in our blood may come from the metabolic processes of the body, but most of it comes from outside sources. In most cases of poisoning the carbon monoxide is produced by the incomplete combustion of carbon producing substances. Important sources are household fuels and automobile exhaust.

Probably the heaviest nonindustrial exposure to carbon monoxide occurs in smokers. The average level of carboxyhemoglobin (carbon monoxide attached to hemoglobin) in persons smoking one pack of cigarettes per day is about 5 percent, in contrast to 1 percent in nonsmokers. A person smoking up to three packs a day may have values of up to 9 percent. As we discussed in Chapter 2 the need for oxygen in the mother-to-be is greater than that in nonpregnant women. This makes the reduced oxygen levels in maternal smokers of added significance.

A recent study at a hospital in Quebec province suggested that some infants born there may have "smoked" half a pack of cigarettes just prior to being born. Thirty-three percent of patients who smoked during pregnancy continued to do so during labor. These women smoked an average of 5.2 cigarettes during labor, with the last one being put out only 3.5 hours before delivery.

Carboxyhemoglobin levels were measured in both smoking and nonsmoking mothers during pregnancy and labor and in the infants right after birth. Carboxyhemoglobin levels in the blood of women who smoked during pregnancy were found to be three times higher than were found in women who did not smoke. This is enough to impair the normal mechanism of the transport of oxygen and lead to a low supply of oxygen to the fetus.

Like nicotine, carbon monoxide crosses the placenta. In

fact, at delivery the level of carboxyhemoglobin in the baby is nearly twice the level found in the mother. This high amount in the circulatory system of the fetus comes about because of two factors. First, the hemoglobin in the baby's blood has a stronger tendency to capture the carbon monoxide than does the hemoglobin in the mother's blood. Second, the carbon monoxide lasts considerably longer in the fetal circulatory system compared to the mother's. The implication of these two differences between the mother and the unborn baby is that for every cigarette smoked by the mother, the fetus gets the equivalent effects of two.

Besides nicotine and carbon monoxide other constituents of smoke may play a role in certain aspects of nutrition. Cigarettes are known to contain small amounts of cyanide and it has been proposed that this compound may affect the ability of the mother to store vitamin B-12, which plays a role in controlling certain types of anemia. During pregnancy, levels of this vitamin are lower in women who smoke than they are in nonsmokers.

Vitamin C is also found to be reduced among pregnant smokers when compared to nonsmokers. As this vitamin is very important for growth of the fetus—in fact, it is recommended that a supplement of this vitamin be taken during pregnancy—its reduction by smoking is an area of high priority for future research.

In subsequent chapters we will examine in detail the variety of possible effects of maternal smoking that we have touched on here. We will also consider the mechanisms by which they may come about and, wherever possible, specify what constituents of cigarette smoke may be playing a role.

chapter four
Mother's Weight Gain during Pregnancy

During a normal pregnancy the mother-to-be goes through a large number of anatomical and physiological changes that affect almost every function of the body. The alterations that occur produce the optimum possible environment for the developing baby. One major change and certainly the most visible is the weight gain of the mother.

All healthy women gain weight during pregnancy. A few, because of morning sickness, do lose weight in the early weeks of pregnancy, but they more than catch up in the later period of gestation. There is considerable variability among individuals in terms of the total number of pounds gained during pregnancy. Young mothers and mothers having a first baby usually gain more than older mothers and women who have had several children. An average range for most healthy mothers-to-be is twenty-four to thirty pounds, although normal births can occur with weight gains ranging from very few to about sixty pounds.

More important than the actual pounds that a woman puts on is the rate of gain and the rate of growth of different systems during pregnancy. Typically during the first trimester the mother gains about two to four pounds. After the third month about a pound a week is the average gain. Table 4-1 shows an approximation of the weight gain during various stages of pregnancy and also how the increase in pounds

Table 4-1.

Approximate Weight Gain in Various Tissues and Systems
during a Normal Pregnancy

Tissues or systems	10 weeks	20 weeks	30 weeks	Term
Fetus	less than 1 oz	3/4 lb	3 1/2 lbs	7 1/2 lbs
Placenta	less than 1 oz	1/3 lb	1 lb	1 1/2 lbs
Amniotic fluid	1 oz	1/2 lb	1 1/3 lbs	1 3/4 lbs
Increase in				
Uterus	1/3 lb	1 1/4 lbs	2 lbs	2 1/2 lbs
Breasts	1 oz	1/2 lb	1 lb	3 lbs
Mother's blood	4 oz	1 1/3 lbs	3 lbs	3 1/2 lbs
Maternal stores	1 lb	4 lbs	6 lbs	7 lbs
Total gain	1 1/2 lbs	9 lbs	18 lbs	27 lbs

is distributed among different systems in the mother, placenta, and fetus.

At the end of the pregnancy the fetus, amniotic fluid (the bag of liquid in which the baby lies), placenta, uterus, and breasts account for about sixteen pounds. The remaining nine to twelve pounds represent an increase in total body water, as well as stored protein and fat. These nutrient reserves are preparation for the growth needs of the fetus during the last ten weeks of gestation and provide the additional energy that will be called upon during labor, birth, and breastfeeding.

During the first ten weeks the mother-to-be typically observes only a small increase in her weight. Much of the gain is caused by the growth of the uterus and the increased blood volume. The fetus at this stage weighs less than an ounce. However, by the end of pregnancy the rapidly growing baby accounts for the largest proportion of the weight gain.

Up to a few years ago much effort was expended by physicians to convince their pregnant patients to restrict their weight gain by reducing the intake of food. This advice was based on the mistaken belief that excessive weight gain is the cause of a serious condition in pregnancy whose symptoms include high blood pressure, a sudden accumulation and retention of fluid in the body tissues making them puffy, and, sometimes, damage to the kidneys. Today it is known that patients with this condition—termed toxemia of pregnancy or preeclampsia—do gain an excessive amount of weight because of fluid retention and not because of overeating.

Accordingly, the practice of severe restriction of diet during pregnancy is carried on no longer. But the pendulum may have swung a little too far in the opposite direction. Although there is ample evidence that a gain of twenty-four to thirty pounds produces the most favorable outcome, and this sort of gain will not occur if food intake is deliberately reduced, the suggestion that pregnant women should "eat to appetite" can be misleading. The mother-to-be must not interpret this advice to mean that she can eat whatever empty calories, or "junk food," she may desire, perhaps justifying this behavior by arguing that whatever the fetus needs, she as a pregnant woman will instinctively crave and eat.

In general, the appetite increases during pregnancy, probably mirroring the need for additional food. There is probably also an emotional basis to the desire to eat as occasionally somewhat unusual tastes are exhibited, with the mother-to-be having an overwhelming urge to eat unusual foods such as pickles and ice cream.

While the old saying that a pregnant woman must eat for two does not express an exact mathematical formula, the need for additional food during pregnancy is real. The increased demand amounts to some two hundred calories per day above the usual diet. However, the total intake is not the critical factor. Rather, the mother-to-be should be concerned with the quality of the food and insure that her diet is balanced and includes the proteins, vitamins, and minerals necessary for the building of tissue, as well as enough energy input from calories to do the work.

There has been considerable interest in determining the relationship between smoking and weight gain of mothers during pregnancy. The primary reason for focusing attention on this issue is to establish the role of maternal weight gain in the widely reported and best known effect of smoking and pregnancy—that babies of smoking mothers generally weigh less at birth than babies of nonsmoking mothers. This relationship between birth weight and smoking will be dealt with in Chapter 5 but here we want to talk about the mother's weight gain during pregnancy, how it may be reflected in the weight of the baby, and how and whether smoking affects maternal weight gain. It seems reasonable to ask whether women who smoke during pregnancy may have a reduced appetite, eat less, and consequently gain less weight, resulting in smaller babies. As we have noted, the relationship between the size of the fetus and the weight gain of the mother during pregnancy changes as pregnancy proceeds. At just over two months the fetus accounts for less than 1 percent of maternal weight gain, but between the tenth and twentieth weeks, 9 percent of the mother's gain represents fetal weight and between the twentieth and thirtieth weeks, the contribution of the fetus increases to 28 percent. During the final ten weeks of the pregnancy almost half of the maternal weight gain is accounted for by the fetus. So, as the pregnancy moves into its later stages the weight of the mother on the bathroom scale is closely tied to the size of the baby inside her.

The evidence relating smoking during pregnancy to maternal weight gain does not present a clear picture. A number of studies have found consistently lower maternal weight gain—averaging 8 percent lower—among smokers compared to nonsmokers. It is proposed that this difference reflects a reduction in appetite and thus in food intake. As indicated by the figures above, the weight gain of the mother during pregnancy and especially during the last few months is closely related to the growth of the fetus. Therefore, it is argued by some that if the mother-to-be eats less, the growth of the fetus may be impeded. If this association between the mother's eating habits and the size of the developing fetus is correct, it has important implications. It suggests that the effects of maternal smoking upon the fetus—or at least some of the effects—may not be direct but rather reflect the cigarettes' influence on the mother. That is, smoking may reduce the mother's food intake and thereby, in an indirect fashion, contribute to a smaller fetus. By following this line of reasoning it then becomes reasonable to propose that some of the effects of cigarette smoking during pregnancy may be eliminated by diet supplementation. This has a popular appeal as it ought to be easier to convince a mother to increase and improve her food intake than to persuade her to give up cigarette smoking. A controlled study examining the possible ameliorative effects of food supplements for smoking mothers has not been carried out, but it certainly would be of considerable interest and importance.

Indirectly supporting the point of view that smoking does not have a major direct effect upon the growth of the fetus but rather exerts its influence on the food intake of the mother is a recent study of over six thousand women. In this work it was reported that on average the weights of regular smoking women before they became pregnant were lower than those of habitual nonsmokers. Furthermore, the weight gain between pregnancies was greater for the nonsmokers than for the habitual smokers. In this sample of six thousand women height did not differ between smokers and non-smokers and therefore the variations in weight probably reflect differences in fatty tissue.

Not all investigators agree with this nutritional interpretation of how smoking affects fetal growth. Some workers have suggested that smoking during pregnancy has a number of independent, direct effects on the mother-to-be, as well as separate effects on the fetus, including the slowing of fetal growth. In other words, maternal smoking results in a *direct* lessening of fetal weight gain. As described earlier, late in the pregnancy the fetus represents a significant proportion of the weight gained by the mother. According to the notion that smoking directly affects fetal size, the mother who smokes may gain less weight during the last few months of pregnancy *because* the fetus is putting on less weight and not the other way around (that is, the fetus is smaller because the smoking mother is not gaining at a normal rate).

This dilemma is a classic example of the difficulty in attributing particular effects to smoking. It is similar to the old chicken and egg problem—which came first? Do some mothers who smoke fail to gain the normal amount during pregnancy because fetal growth is slowed or is the fetus smaller because of the effect smoking has upon food intake in some mothers?

To complicate the issue further, a number of researchers have reported no differences in weight gain during pregnancy between smokers and nonsmokers. One can find about the same number of scientists on both sides of the fence. There is no readily apparent reason for the inconsistent findings. Factors such as socioeconomic level, general health, the number of previous pregnancies, nutritional habits, and use of other drugs such as alcohol have been eliminated as causes of the different findings of the various researchers.

For example, in a German study that involved over six thousand pregnant women no differences in weight gain among nonsmokers, light smokers, and heavy smokers were observed, yet there was a clear relationship between the amount smoked and the degree of reduction of birth weight in the newborns. A very similar trend emerged from examining the records of over thirty thousand Canadian mothers and their babies. Maternal weight gain was the same for nonsmokers and smokers but birth weights differed.

It is apparent that at this time we are in a quandary with respect to the question of smoking and the effect it may have upon the weight gain of the mother-to-be. Nearly all possible results have been reported. Several studies have found no reduction in the weight gain of smoking pregnant women;

others have found some reduction and have attributed it to diminished food intake; and others who have found a reduced maternal weight gain have attributed this phenomenon to a direct reduction by smoking of fetal growth. Clearly, this is an issue that remains to be resolved.

chapter five
The Placenta

The placenta, or afterbirth, is a flat, spongy organ that lies in the cavity of the uterus, attached to the uterine wall. In appearance the placenta is similar to a pancake, which is what the Latin word it derives from means. By the end of pregnancy it measures seven inches in diameter and one inch in thickness. As a rule, the weight of the placenta is one-sixth that of the baby; since the average newborn infant weighs seven to seven and a half pounds, the typical placental weight is one and a quarter pounds.

The vital role that the placenta plays as a link between mother and child is anatomically very clear. The placenta has two sides. One is in contact with the wall of the uterus and the other faces the fetus. The maternal side is deep red in color and is divided into sections that fit into depressed areas in the wall of the uterus and are attached there. The fetal side is smooth and shiny and projects into the cavity of the uterus. The umbilical cord, the lifeline that connects the placenta and the fetus, is attached to this side.

The placenta makes its appearance and starts its life-sustaining functions very early in embryonic development. At ovulation the egg is discharged from the ovary and enters the Fallopian tube. There are two Fallopian tubes, one on each side of the pelvic cavity, extending from the upper part of the uterus to the ovary. The egg passes along the tube toward the uterus. It is in the tube that the egg meets the sperm, is fertilized, and begins to divide. During the time it is in the tube the fertilized egg undergoes considerable development. The actual size does not increase a great deal but the number of cells does and while it is in the Fallopian tube the fertilized ovum (egg) is a solid mass of cells. By the fifth or sixth day after ovulation the egg reaches the interior of the uterus. It remains unattached, in a free-floating state, for twenty-four hours or more.

The next phase is that of implantation. Under the stimulation of the ovarian hormones the inner lining of the uterus has undergone special preparation to receive the fertilized egg. The lining becomes thicker and spongier, and the egg, which has been lying unattached in the cavity of the uterus, proceeds to burrow its way into this lining. By seven and a half days after ovulation this process of implantation is complete. The egg lies entirely within the wall of the uterus, although a small bulge over the surface remains.

The growing and developing egg contains within itself only a limited amount of nutrients so that within a short time it must obtain oxygen and food from other sources. To this end the cells that form the outer layer of the embryo develop a special function. They make contact with the small spaces in the uterus that are filled with blood, extract food and oxygen from the maternal blood, and pass these substances along to the other cells of the embryo. These special cells function as a primitive placenta and begin their work as early as the eleventh day following ovulation.

Because its aim is to make as close a contact as possible with maternal blood, the placenta is typically located in the area of the uterus in which the supply of blood is most abundant. The cells of the primitive placenta send rootlike projections known as villi into the mother's uterus, where they lie bathed in small pools of blood. The villi themselves contain blood vessels that connect to the fetal circulatory system via the umbilical cord. This arrangement results in maternal blood on the outside of the placental villi and the baby's blood on the inside. There is no mixing of maternal and fetal blood supplies: the blood of the mother does not enter the circulatory system of the fetus, nor does that of the fetus enter the mother's bloodstream. The exchange of nourishment, oxygen, and waste products between the blood supply of the mother and that of fetus takes place across the thin walls of the villi.

How well the placenta performs its function is one of the critical determinations of fetal well-being. If the villi are reduced in size or number or if there is an insufficient network of blood vessels, the supply of oxygen and food may be insufficient to allow for the normal growth of the fetus.

The placenta has two main fields of activity. First, it acts as a route of transfer; it is the only communication between mother and child. Second, the placenta is a sophisticated factory, taking substances from both the mother and the fetus, breaking them down into simple compounds, and then manufacturing new and complicated products. Some of these go to the fetus and others to the mother. One thing that the placenta is unable to do, however, is to recognize and reject substances that are harmful to the fetus; thus, anything that circulates in the maternal blood has the potential of crossing the placenta and reaching the fetus. It is thought that any substance found in the maternal or fetal blood can cross the placenta to some extent unless it is destroyed or altered during passage. What the placenta may do however is to greatly slow down the rate at which substances can cross from mother to fetus. In some cases the placenta's low degree of permeability results in certain substances crossing to the fetus at such a low rate that essentially they have little physiological effect. The term "placental barrier" signifies the role of the placenta as an organ for the controlled transfer of materials rather than that of an organ that merely obstructs the passage of certain substances.

For the fetus in utero the placenta performs many functions that are taken over by specific organs after birth. For example, the placenta plays the role of the lungs. In the adult the lungs are composed of numerous small air sacs that are richly supplied with blood vessels. Oxygen, as well as other constituents of inspired (or inhaled) air, passes from the air sacs into the bloodstream. Carbon dioxide passes from the bloodstream into the air sacs and is excreted into the air by the process of expiration (or exhalation).

An analogy has been made between the function of the lungs and that of the placenta, especially in regard to the transfer of oxygen and carbon dioxide. In both organs this activity is critical since even a brief deficiency in the amount and speed of passage of oxygen can have very serious consequences. A significant difference between the two is that in the placenta the exchange of the respiratory gases is from blood to blood, while in the lungs it is from air to blood. In the lungs the process is one of passive diffusion in response to differences of concentration; in the placenta, as has been described, the process for many substances is much more complicated.

The placenta acts as the fetal kidney, removing the waste products from the infant and excreting them by way of the maternal bloodstream. Failure of the placenta in this action would have the same serious effects as failure of the kidneys in the adult.

The liver is the largest gland in the body. Among its numerous activities is the secretion of bile. The liver acts as an energy storehouse by extracting glucose (sugar) from the blood and converting it to glycogen, which it stores. When the need arises, the glycogen is converted back to glucose, which is then used for the production of energy. The liver also converts the waste products of the digestion of protein into a form that the kidneys can eliminate, and it detoxifies poisonous substances so that they become harmless.

The placenta has certain similarities to the liver in that it is an amazingly diverse organ that manufactures enormous and varied amounts of enzymes and hormones essential to the well-being of the fetus. More than sixty enzymes have been detected in the placenta.

One important enzymatic action mediated by the placenta involves oxytocinase. Oxytocin is a substance produced by a part of the brain known as the hypothalamus; oxytocin is stored in a gland—the pituitary—that is attached to the base of the brain. When released into the bloodstream, oxytocin has the effect of inducing uterine contractions. At the end of pregnancy, when the fetus is mature, this is a normal event. In the early part of pregnancy a high level of oxytocin might bring on premature labor. Normally the oxytocinase produced by the placenta destroys the oxytocin. Should the placenta fail to produce adequate amounts of oxytocinase, the oxytocin would be unopposed and labor might begin before the baby is ready for the outside world.

It is clear that the placenta plays a role of enormous importance. Interference with its multifaceted functioning may disrupt the well-being of the fetus.

Tobacco smoke, with its most active constituent, nicotine, is inhaled into the lungs, from there is absorbed into the bloodstream of the mother, and makes its way throughout the body, including, in pregnant women, the placenta. Nicotine, regardless of its possible effects on the uterus and the placenta, is a substance that crosses the placenta freely and enters the fetal circulation.

From the description of the preceding pages it is clear that the placenta is a marvelously complex organ with numerous functions vital to the life and growth of the developing fetus. Because in smoking mothers-to-be the placenta is exposed to constituents of tobacco, it is of considerable importance whether smoking affects the organ itself and its functions.

Early in the second trimester of pregnancy the size of the placenta is about equal to that of the fetus. Although the placenta continues to grow until the latter part of the pregnancy, it does not keep up with the fetus. At term the weight of the placenta is about one-sixth that of the fetus, as we noted earlier. In order to be able to nourish the growing fetus the placenta must increase both its size and its function. Several studies have been carried out to determine whether or not the weight of the placenta differs between smokers and nonsmokers. Some workers have found no difference in the mean placental weight between women who smoke and those who do not. Others claim that the placenta is smaller in smokers and a few investigators have noted that placental size is increased slightly in women who smoke heavily. The explanation of this last finding is that the placenta becomes larger to compensate for the reduced oxygen level in the blood of women who smoke. The implications of this possibility will be considered in Chapter 7 when we examine the size of the placenta in terms of its being a ratio of the size of the fetus.

Investigations of placental circulation have shown that smoking even one standard cigarette causes an immediate, short-term decrease in the flow of blood in the portion of the uterus in which the villi lie and from which they obtain the substances that the fetus needs. It is known that nicotine causes a temporary narrowing of the uterine blood vessels, leading to a reduction in the amount of blood flowing through the uterus and the placenta. This effect disappears within fifteen minutes after smoking has ceased. It is possible that this temporary decrease in the flow of blood, if it occurs repeatedly, may, by leading to a reduction in the supply of oxygen and food to the fetus, be responsible for some of the effects seen in infants born to smoking mothers. These effects will be discussed in the next few chapters.

The reduction in uterine blood flow and the decrease in oxygen available to the fetus take on added significance when one recalls our earlier discussion of the effects of carbon monoxide, which is produced by the burning of tobacco. The carbon monoxide attaches itself to the hemoglobin on red blood cells and, by doing so, reduces the ability of the hemoglobin to carry out its normal function of transporting oxygen. This means that the mother-to-be who smokes may be reducing the amount of oxygen available to the fetus in two ways that add together—a reduced blood flow and a decreased capacity of the blood to carry oxygen.

One way of assessing the effects upon the placenta of smoking is by comparing the frequencies of complications during pregnancy between smokers and nonsmokers. These results are presented in detail in Chapter 6. The overall picture is that among smokers there is an increased incidence of premature separation of the placenta from the wall of the uterus, bleeding during pregnancy, and possibly spontaneous abortions. These results clearly indicate that the use of cigarettes by the pregnant woman increases the probability of placental malfunctioning and distress on the part of the unborn baby.

chapter six

Complications during Pregnancy

Is maternal smoking associated with an increased risk of very serious and possibly fatal complications during pregnancy? This is the central issue of this chapter.

The methods used to examine the possible linkage between smoking and problems during pregnancy are similar to those used to establish whether particular substances will cause complications during pregnancy. It is not an easy task. Two general approaches are taken by researchers. One method consists of making extensive inquiries after the complications have been diagnosed. This procedure is termed retrospective research, as the possible causes are sought after the identification of the problem. Typically this sort of research relies on the mother's recollection of what she did or did not do during different stages of her pregnancy and on medical records. In both cases relevant details may not be available or may have been forgotten or overlooked.

Retrospective studies can vary tremendously in scope. A few have been carried out on a huge scale. For example, in Great Britain in 1958 virtually all the births occurring during a particular week were carefully monitored and questionnaires given to over seventeen thousand mothers. In another instance, data were collected for over fifty thousand births and fetal deaths that occurred in ten hospitals during a one-year period in Ontario. In large surveys such as these an enormous mass of information is collected and recorded in great detail and can, in some cases, be a useful step in determining the underlying causes of complications during pregnancy. Obviously, however, such a thorough approach is a prodigious undertaking and most retrospective studies are not of that scale nor, as a consequence, are they as informative.

A second approach used by investigators, and in fact utilized in our own ongoing work described in the introduction, is termed the prospective procedure. This technique involves the recording of information from expectant mothers before any complications have been observed. If problems then occur during the pregnancy an attempt is made to see whether any association between the previously acquired information and the complication can be made. The principal advantage of this procedure is that the information collected during the pregnancy does not rely on memory. There are, however, serious difficulties with the prospective approach. When information is collected during pregnancy before any problems have arisen, what facts are to be recorded? As one does not know beforehand what is going to be relevant, a large amount of unnecessary information may be gathered or, more serious, some critical details may not be obtained. An additional difficulty is that as there is no way to predict who is going to have complications during pregnancy and as complications occur relatively infrequently, a large number of expectant women have to be involved.

Whether a retrospective or a prospective approach is used, the determination as to whether a particular substance may increase the likelihood of complications during pregnancy involves a comparison between two groups of women. First, the rate of occurrence of problems during pregnancy in women who are exposed to the substance in question is determined. Then, this rate is contrasted to that found among mothers-to-be who are not exposed to the same substance. The differences between the groups is described as the risk factor for the substance in question.

However, in order to be sure that the risk to the baby is in fact posed by the factor being examined and not some other factor, the expectant mothers in one group must be similar to the women in the other group in as many characteristics as possible. When examining the issue of smoking this comparability between the groups is of considerable importance. A few examples will serve to highlight this problem.

Several studies have shown that the risk of complications during pregnancy rises after two babies. Also, after several pregnancies the likelihood that the expectant mother smokes increases. In other words, women pregnant for the first time are less likely to be smokers than pregnant women who already have several children. Another point to mention here is that first-time mothers who do smoke tend to be light smokers. So, if we were to divide expectant mothers into two groups solely on the basis of whether or not they smoked during pregnancy, it is likely that in the nonsmoker (and light smoker) group there would be more first-time mothers-to-be than in the smoker group. And, continuing this line of reasoning, women with more than two babies would be more likely to be found in the smoking group than in the nonsmoking group. Since the likelihood of prenatal complications increases in women after the second pregnancy and as there may be more of these women in the smoking group than the nonsmoking group, a confusing situation results. How does one separate out the risk factor that may arise from cigarettes from the risk factor associated with multiple pregnancies. Obviously, then, it is important to take into account the number of previous pregnancies in the smoking and nonsmoking groups.

A second example that indicates the importance of comparability between smoking and nonsmoking groups in as many respects as possible except for the cigarette habit can be seen when considering racial and economic background. In the British Isles more women in the lower socioeconomic class smoke than do those in other social classes. Also associated with the lower social category are increased complications during pregnancy. Thus, in Great Britain, the division of expectant mothers into smokers and nonsmokers may also result in an uneven distribution of women in terms of socioeconomic class. In the smoking group, therefore, the risk factor associated with cigarette use may be compounded by the risk factor associated with the lower social class. In the United States complications during pregnancy have a greater probability of occurring among black mothers-to-be than among white mothers. But the incidence of smoking during pregnancy and the number of cigarettes smoked are greater among whites. If one ignored racial background when dividing women into smokers and nonsmokers, there would tend to be more nonsmokers from the higher risk black racial group and more smokers from the lower risk white racial group. Thus, the two factors of race and smoking may cancel each other out.

These two examples illustrate how easy it is to draw false conclusions from data that on the surface appear quite clear-cut. Errors can be made in both directions. In one case effects may be attributed to smoking when in reality other factors may be playing a critical role. On the other hand, no effect may be seen when in fact the possible role of smoking is masked or hidden by the makeup of the groups being considered.

There is considerable controversy as to whether smoking during pregnancy increases the risk of fetal death. The reason for the uncertainty lies in the fact that fetal mortality can occur in different ways and each of these ways is influenced by different factors that may or may not interact with smoking. For example, spontaneous abortion may arise from infections or from an imbalance of hormones. On the other hand, stillbirths may be caused by, among other factors, the premature separation of the placenta from the wall of the uterus. Some studies have examined the relationship between various types of fetal death and smoking whereas others have lumped together all forms of fetal mortality and smoking. Given this mixed approach it is perhaps not surprising that no clear-cut picture has emerged.

Many researchers have reported that the rate of spontaneous abortion is higher among smokers than among nonsmokers. Moreover, according to the findings of a number of investigators, the incidence increases as the amount smoked during pregnancy goes up. Work done in the 1960s found that the percentage of spontaneous abortions was about 12.5 percent among smokers and just under 9 percent among nonsmokers. The significance of these findings, however, is not clear for a number of reasons. Virtually all of the studies undertaken prior to 1970 did not make allowance for variables other than cigerette smoking that may influence the rate of spontaneous abortion. Included among these would be the age of the mother, the general health of the woman, the number of previous pregnancies, and whether the pregnancy was a wanted one. One may wonder about the relevance of a wanted pregnancy and smoking. Surprisingly, this factor was found to be of considerable importance in a Swedish study reported in 1971 that involved over six thousand pregnancies. The Scandinavian researchers noted that the likelihood of spontaneous abortion approximately doubled in unwanted pregnancies. The workers also noted that more of the smokers' than the nonsmokers' pregnancies were unwanted. After comparing the number of spontaneous abortions that occurred in smoking and nonsmoking women, an increased risk was found among the smokers but this relationship to a considerable degree reflected the association between smoking and unwanted pregnancy.

A recent study that took into account such factors as age, previous pregnancies, and previous abortions reported that spontaneous abortions occurred almost twice as frequently among smokers compared to among nonsmokers. The fact that this work separated the risk associated with smoking from other influencing variables suggests that smoking during pregnancy is a risk factor for spontaneous abortion. But until more data are in, firm conclusions cannot be drawn.

The relationship of cigarettes and stillbirth is somewhat clearer than that between smoking and spontaneous abortion. Yet the first investigations in this area in the 1960s were almost evenly divided between those reporting more stillbirths among smokers than among nonsmokers and those that found no differences. Factors such as age of the mother or number of other births did not seem to explain the apparently discrepant findings.

Recent studies have shed considerable light both on the issue of smoking and stillbirth and on the inconsistency of earlier findings. Studies undertaken in the 1970s have generally found that among white women stillbirths do not appear to be associated with smoking. However, among blacks a relationship between smoking and stillbirths was observed, with the increase in the number of fetal deaths being greater among the heavier smokers. Although there are many possible interpretations of these results, most researchers believe that the difference between the races is based on socioeconomic factors. In general, the economic and social conditions of the black family are not as favorable as those experienced by whites. This difference is felt to underlie, at least in part, the fact that even among nonsmokers stillbirths occur more often among black women than among white. What is particularly important here, however, is that this difference increases when a comparison is made between women of the two races who smoked during pregnancy. Basically what happens is that among whites smoking does not alter the likelihood of stillbirth but among blacks smoking does. In other words, the combination of smoking and a relatively poor socioeconomic environment has a markedly greater effect on the chance of stillbirth than the combination of smoking and a more favorable socioeconomic level. The unfavorable socioeconomic situation is itself a risk factor as far as stillbirths are concerned. Combining this variable with smoking adds to the risk factor. This additive relationship between smoking and other risk factors appears to be a general one when considering stillbirths. Women who for one reason or another can be described as having a pregnancy that is at some risk increase this risk by smoking and do so to a greater degree than smokers who do not have the initial reproductive risk during pregnancy.

Overall, then, in particular circumstances, maternal smoking does appear to increase the risk of fetal death. It must be pointed out, however, that in absolute numbers the increased incidence of fetal deaths is small. For example, a study conducted in Wales found 130 stillbirths per 10,000 births among nonsmokers as compared to 154 stillbirths per 10,000 births among smokers. In a Canadian study the rate among nonsmokers was 110 per 10,000 births whereas among smokers it was 140 per 10,000 births. Although in terms of numbers the difference between smokers and nonsmokers is relatively slight, the increased risk expressed in percentages is striking: the smoker has an 18 to 36 percent (depending on which study is used) greater likelihood than a nonsmoker of having a pregnancy terminate in a stillbirth.

The exact route by which cigarette smoking may affect the unborn cannot be specified but there are three likely ways. The first is a relatively indirect mechanism. It involves changes in the expectant mother's biological functions such as altered breathing and heart rates, which in turn may have an effect on the fetus. A more direct mechanism by which the products of smoking, such as nicotine and carbon monoxide, may affect the fetus is by altering the rate at which oxygen and nutrients cross the placenta from the mother to the unborn baby. Finally, the expectant mother's smoking habit can affect the fetus by a direct diffusion mechanism through the placenta. That is, the by-products of smoking present in the mother's bloodstream may themselves cross the placenta, enter the circulatory system of the fetus, and act directly on the developing baby.

In instances in which smoking has played a contributory role in the death of a fetus the direct cause is thought to be an inadequate supply of oxygen. Before birth the baby is entirely dependent upon the mother for oxygen. As the fetus has no direct access to air, all the oxygen needed to survive and grow is obtained from the mother's blood. The mechanism for the transfer of oxygen from mother to child is quite straightforward. The surface of the placenta is bathed by a pool of the mother's blood that is carrying oxygen. This oxygen leaves the mother's blood supply, crosses the placental wall, and enters the bloodstream of the baby. It is not necessary for the two bloodstreams to be in direct contact for this transfer of oxygen to take place. Once the oxygen enters the circulatory system of the baby, the fetal heart pumps the blood from the placenta, along the umbilical cord, and into the baby's tissues.

All living tissue or, more precisely, the cells making up the tissue require oxygen to live. Shortages of this life-sustaining element can result in death. Such oxygen deficiencies can occur in any or all of the three different but intertwined systems—the mother, the placenta, and the fetus.

Earlier we stated that a deficiency of oxygen is the suspected immediate cause of many fetal deaths associated with smoking. This is, in a sense, somewhat misleading. When an elderly person dies, frequently the direct or immediate cause of death is pneumonia. Usually, however, some other condition such as the flu actually precipitated the pneumonia. In the case of the unborn baby and oxygen deprivation a parallel situation exists. Although an oxygen shortage is the likely immediate cause of death, in many cases placental complications appear to be the precipitating factor. The complications can take a variety of forms, as described at the beginning of this chapter. Two particular placental problems appear to be more prevalent among smokers than nonsmokers: placenta previa (a condition in which the placenta lies over the cervix and in front of the fetus, blocking the passage) and abruptio placenta (premature separation, either partial or complete, of the placenta from the wall of the uterus).

Some researchers think that smoking may contribute to these potentially serious placental complications by reducing the oxygen level in the fetal blood. If this is the case an unfortunate chain reaction comes into play. Smoking causes a moderate reduction in the oxygen carried to the fetus. This deficit in turn may disrupt normal placental-fetal communication and result in a potentially fatal oxygen depletion in the unborn baby's system.

Cigarette smoking by the mother-to-be can reduce the oxygenation of the fetal blood in a number of ways. One of the products of smoking is nicotine, which causes blood vessels to become smaller in diameter. This narrowing of the passages through which the blood passes decreases the blood supply through the placenta and thus reduces the oxygen going from the mother to the unborn baby. This lowered rate of flow is short lasting, the flow returning to normal a few minutes after smoking has stopped. However, the effects of the repeated reduction of blood flowing from the uterus to the placenta that would occur with regular smoking have not been determined and they may contribute to the placental complications described earlier.

Another direct way in which smoking may reduce the oxygen available to the tissues of the fetus is by the accumulation of carbon monoxide. As described in Chapter 2, carbon monoxide combines with a substance in the blood called hemoglobin to produce carboxyhemoglobin. This combination of carbon monoxide with hemoglobin reduces the ability of hemoglobin to do its normal job, that is, to

55

pick up, transport, and deposit oxygen. This lowering of the oxygen function of the hemoglobin occurs in both the mother and the fetus. In fact, as we have noted, the level of carboxyhemoglobin in the fetus is almost twice as high as that found in the mother at any particular time, indicating that carbon monoxide appears to accumulate in the fetus. Carbon monoxide has an additional effect. The hemoglobin in the blood that has not combined with carbon monoxide is still capable of carrying oxygen, but the presence of carbon monoxide hinders the hemoglobin from giving up the oxygen it is carrying to the tissues that need it. Thus, carbon monoxide has a dual effect, both of which reduce oxygen availability: it lessens the capacity of the blood to carry oxygen and it hampers the release into tissues of the oxygen that is available from the blood.

As indicated earlier, some workers argue that these lowered oxygen levels may be a contributing factor to the placental complications associated with smoking. Although the amount of carboxyhemoglobin may prove to have some bearing on the incidence of fetal death, other mechanisms also play an important role in linking smoking and stillbirth. In a community in India tobacco chewing (as contrasted to smoking) is quite common, occurring among approximately 16 percent of pregnant women. The women keep a wad of tobacco in the mouth for eight to ten hours a day, renewing the wad hourly. The amount of nicotine placed in the mouth is enormous—as high as four grams a day, roughly equivalent to the nicotine contained in over four thousand cigarettes. Obviously, only a very small percentage of the chewed nicotine enters the woman's system. How much, however, has not been ascertained. By chewing rather than smoking the tobacco no carbon monoxide is formed and thus observations of complications during pregnancy can be attributed to factors other than altered hemoglobin. The stillbirth rate of those who chewed tobacco was fifty per thousand; among women who did not chew tobacco the rate was seventeen per thousand. The figure for nonusers is quite similar to the stillbirth rates of nonsmokers in North America and Europe cited earlier in this chapter. However, among tobacco users a much more dramatic increase in the rate of stillbirth was noted among those who chewed tobacco contrasted to those who smoked cigarettes. It is likely that the high quantity of nicotine is the major contributing factor in the almost 300 percent increase in stillbirths among those who chewed tobacco. However, until the nicotine levels in the blood are determined, the role that this substance is playing cannot be specified.

Interestingly, there is one particular form of complication observed during pregnancy that is found less often among smokers than among nonsmokers. This condition, termed preeclampsia, occurs late in pregnancy and as we noted earlier it is characterized by rising blood pressure, possible kidney failure, and an accumulation of fluid in tissues, giving them a puffy appearance. There is also a thickening of the placental wall, making it more difficult for oxygen to diffuse from the mother to the unborn baby. If the expectant mother is not treated, she may experience severe convulsions. A number of doctors attribute this lowered incidence of preeclampsia to one of the constituents found in the blood of cigarette users. This substance is thiocyanate, which is a product of cyanide (the same poison so frequently used in who-dun-it books), a constituent of cigarette smoke. Thiocyanate reduces blood pressure and this effect is thought to reduce the likelihood of preeclampsia.

Several scientific reports indicate that the association between smoking and the risk of fetal death does not remain constant throughout pregnancy. Although the probability of risk to the fetus is greater among smokers than among nonsmokers throughout pregnancy, the biggest difference between the two groups occurs between the twentieth and the thirtieth week. This period during mid-pregnancy is the time of most rapid growth not only in utero but in fact during the person's entire life. (It has been estimated that if the unborn baby kept on growing at this rate, by age fifteen the child would be seventy-five feet tall.)

During this period of maximum growth rate, the developing fetus has increased energy needs and displays a particularly high demand for oxygen. Therefore, the unborn baby at this stage of pregnancy may be especially vulnerable to a diminished oxygen supply; thus, during mid-gestation the most marked differences are observed in fetal risk between smokers and nonsmokers.

Since the Thalidomide tragedy of the early 1960s, in which a sedative prescribed to expectant mothers caused gross malformations particularly in the limbs of the unborn, there has been considerable awareness of the possible severe effects drugs may have on the developing embryo. In the case of cigarettes there is no evidence to suggest that smoking during pregnancy increases the incidence of physical abnormalities in the newborn although some workers, a relative minority, have reported that facial deformities such as cleft palate and harelip are somewhat increased among the infants of smoking mothers.

However, smoking may be an important contributing factor in another category of physical anomalies that are life-threatening. In the United States it has recently been estimated that physical abnormalities of the fetus cause over 9 percent of all deaths of babies during the last half of pregnancy and the first month after birth. This makes such congenital anomalies (for example, defects of the heart) the fourth most common cause of mortality during this time period. In an American study that reviewed over fifty thousand births evidence was gathered that indicated that the rate of congenital abnormalities increased if the mother smoked ten or more cigarettes per day during pregnancy. Moreover, as the woman's cigarette habit increased so did the probability of these abnormalities.

This is one of the very few studies to report evidence

that smoking increases the likelihood of physical defects .
the fetus. The size of the sample examined and the significant
nature of the abnormalities have made this study receive a
lot of attention from both the press and the scientific community. It is a safe prediction that much effort will be
directed at verifying these results.

chapter seven

Fetal Growth, Birth Weight, and Prematurity

North American adults are leading longer and healthier lives but our babies are not doing as well. In the United States the infant death rate is 16.5 out of every 1000 live births and in Canada the rate is 15.0 out of every 1000. These numbers place Canada eleventh in the world in terms of infant mortality and the United States close behind. The vast majority of babies who die before the onset of labor, during labor, or in the first few weeks after birth are of low birth weight (under five and a half pounds, or less than twenty-five hundred grams). In North America approximately 7.5 percent of babies are of low birth weight and have a reduced chance of being completely normal if they do survive.

Babies small at birth may be divided into two groups. In the first are those infants born too soon but whose size is appropriate for the period of gestation. This means that, whatever the duration of the pregnancy may be when the baby is born, the size of the infant is that expected for his or her gestational age, or how long the baby has been carried. These infants are described as being premature or preterm. In the second group are babies who are smaller than average for their gestational age. These children have failed to develop properly in utero. They are small but not necessarily premature. Such children are described as being small for their gestational age or small for dates.

Dated from the time of ovulation or the day of the successful coitus, the gestation period is approximately 266 days. However, since it is rare in human beings to know either the date of ovulation or that of the fertile coitus, the pregnancy is dated from the first day of the last normal menstrual period; the length of the pregnancy is about 280 days (or forty weeks) from this day.

On the basis of the duration of pregnancy when birth occurs, babies have been divided into three groups. A preterm infant is one born when the period of gestation at birth is less than thirty-seven completed weeks (259 days) from the first day of the last menstrual period. A term infant is one born when the period of gestation is from thirty-seven to less than forty-two completed weeks (259 to 293 days) from the first day of the last menstrual period. A postterm infant is one born when the period of gestation is forty-two weeks (294 days) or more from the first day of the last menstrual period.

A premature infant is one born at a stage of pregnancy when the vital organs have not developed to a point where the chances of survival outside the uterus are as good as those of an infant who has had the benefit of a full period of intrauterine growth. The main problem is in the function of the lungs, specifically in their ability to supply the baby with adequate oxygen. Although only 7 to 8 percent of pregnancies terminate before thirty-four weeks, the majority of deaths at or around birth fall into this group.

Premature labor is a high-risk condition for the infant and often for the mother as well. Preterm labor and delivery occur in some 10 to 15 percent of pregnancies in developed countries and more frequently in underdeveloped areas and in socioeconomically deprived populations. In many instances the exact reason for the premature labor is not known.

The outlook for the premature infant is affected by the size at birth. Most newborn babies who weigh more than five and a half pounds have no difficulty in coping with life outside the uterus. On the other hand, infants who weigh under five and a half pounds when they are born do have problems, and these become progressively more serious as the weight falls further below five and a half pounds. The largest number of babies who die in the first twenty-eight days of life weigh less than five and a half pounds at birth.

The short- and long-term outlook for premature infants is much less optimistic than that for full term babies, as the following review indicates. (1) Prematurity is the most common recurring factor in the illnesses and deaths of newborns. (2) As compared with the mature infant the premature baby is more troubled by a variety of conditions: hypoxia (insufficient oxygen) is twelve times, intracranial hemorrhage five times, cerebral palsy ten times, mental deficiency five times, and lethal malformations seven times as frequent. (3) There is a higher incidence of brain damage in premature babies. The soft bones of the skull are less able to protect the immature brain from the compression of the head that occurs during labor and delivery. (4) The respiratory distress syndrome is responsible for many deaths in premature infants. This is a severe disorder of the lungs that is a consequence of the infant's being born before the lungs have reached functional maturity. It affects mainly the preterm baby. Normally, when the infant takes his or her first big breath at birth, the lungs expand and remain partly inflated after most of the air is expired. Subsequent breaths require far less inspiratory effort. The immature lungs cannot hold residual air and collapse with each expiration. The same high inflating pressure is required at the next breath, and again the lungs collapse after expiration. In effect, the baby is taking a first breath again and again and soon becomes exhausted. The transfer of oxygen from the lungs into the infant's circulation is impaired, the baby is in a state of insufficient oxygenation, and his or her condition deteriorates gradually.

Like premature infants, babies of low birth weight are at greater risk than are infants of normal size. To begin with, 10 percent have serious congenital abnormalities, some of which may endanger life. Many of the remainder breathe poorly at birth and require artificial respiration. On occasion a mixture of amniotic fluid and meconium (fetal stool) is sucked into the air passages, preventing oxygen from reaching the air sacs of the lungs. Body temperature and blood sugar level are low, and susceptibility to infection is high.

From the above descriptions it is apparent that babies with a birth weight of under five and a half pounds, whether they be premature or small for dates, run a considerably greater risk of having problems than do larger infants. The relationship of smoking during pregnancy and low birth weight is the most widely written about topic in the general area of cigarettes and pregnancy.

Since the mid-1950s some fifty studies have pursued the question of the relationship between smoking during pregnancy and the growth of the fetus. These investigations have involved a large number of women and babies. A recent count has estimated that the birth weights of over half a million newborns have been measured in this line of research.

The first thorough documentation of a relationship between smoking and birth weight was reported in 1957. In this study a California investigator studied the babies of 7499 women. She noted that infants who at birth weighed less than five and a half pounds were approximately twice as numerous among cigarette smokers as among nonsmokers. Furthermore, the author observed what in scientific terms is called a dose response relationship. That is, the probability of a woman's giving birth to a baby defined as premature (under five and a half pounds) rose as the number of cigarettes smoked daily increased.

Since that initial study there has been a degree of unanimity that is unusual in scientific literature. Virtually all studies have reported that there is a clear relationship between cigarette smoking and lower infant birth weight. Most authors go one step further, a large, important step. They argue that the evidence is such that not only is there an association between maternal smoking and low birth weight but this association is a causal one. In other words, the lower birth weight of babies born to smoking mothers is caused by the cigarette habit during pregnancy.

What is the evidence that has led to this cause and effect interpretation? Many factors besides smoking have been associated with low birth weight, including low socioeconomic status, particular geographic locations, racial or cultural background, age, and number of previous pregnancies. As women who smoke during pregnancy may also fall into one or more of these other risk categories, the problem is one of separating the role of smoking from that of other factors. Because of the enormous number of mothers and infants who have been investigated with respect to maternal smoking habits, it has been possible to do this. Such studies have indicated that regardless of other factors smoking during pregnancy appears to be directly associated with low birth weight.

The fact that numerous researchers have shown a dose relationship between smoking and lowered birth weight adds considerable credence to a cause and effect interpretation. One large study conducted in the early 1960s in Ontario included fifty thousand births. The authors found that the likelihood of a baby's weighing less than five and a half pounds was 70 percent greater than that for nonsmokers if the mother-to-be smoked less than a pack a day. The probability of having a low birth weight infant jumped to 160 percent compared to nonsmokers if the mother smoked more than a pack a day.

An additional convincing argument for identifying a causal relationship between smoking and low birth weight is the finding that if a mother-to-be gives up smoking early in pregnancy her baby will weigh virtually the same as an infant born to a nonsmoker. Finally, in a study reported in 1978, the data from over fifty-three thousand pregnancies indicated that mothers who smoked during one pregnancy but not during another had infants of lower birth weight after the pregnancy in which they had smoked. As indicated earlier in this chapter, five and a half pounds is the clinically accepted borderline used to define a low birth weight baby. But certainly not all babies born to smokers are below this figure. For example, in the Canadian study mentioned above 12 percent of the heavy smokers gave birth to infants in the low birth weight category as contrasted to a 5 percent rate among nonsmokers. Thus, although a woman who smokes during pregnancy increases dramatically the risk of having a low birth weight baby, the vast majority of women who smoke a pack or more per day will not have such an infant. But, even among those women who have babies within the so-called normal range, the likelihood is that the infant will weigh less than a baby born to a nonsmoker. Almost fifty studies came to this conclusion. The average difference in birth weight between smokers and nonsmokers from all these studies is approximately eight ounces, with a clear dose relationship frequently reported as the more marked reduction is observed in those mothers who are the heavier smokers. If an infant is in the normal birth weight range, a reduction of eight ounces is usually not of clinical significance. What might be a more important issue, however, is the question of what are the underlying mechanisms responsible for this growth reduction. For, if the mechanisms are causing a slightly smaller baby might they not also be affecting other, possibly more subtle, aspects of the newborn's physical and mental health?

Some authors propose that in spite of the large number of studies that suggest a cause and effect relationship between smoking and small infants the link is actually only an indirect one. The data upon which this conclusion is based are intriguing. The fundamental first step in this argument is that smokers as a whole are different from nonsmokers in more ways than just their cigarette habit. Few scientific investigators would disagree with this claim. For example, smokers as a group tend to drink more coffee and alcholic beverages than do nonsmokers. The two groups also differ, among other things, in terms of work history, education, and number of previous pregnancies. As mentioned earlier, when factors that are known to influence or are suspected of influencing birth weight are considered, smoking during pregnancy still has its own demonstrable effect. But those who do not accept a direct causal effect of smoking argue that what is really being observed in these and a multitude of other studies are the effects of the *smoker* as opposed to the effects of *smoking.* The investigation that served as the basis for this interpretation was reported in the early 1970s. It involved questioning over five thousand women about their smoking habits during and after previous pregnancies. The researchers found that low birth weight occurred as often in babies born to mothers who started smoking after pregnancy as in babies whose mothers smoked during pregnancy. In other words, women who became smokers had newborns who did not differ in weight from babies born to smoking mothers. These results appear to argue against the notion that cigarette smoking is a direct causal element in the higher incidence of low birth weight and implies that the smaller baby appears to reflect some characteristics of the smoker herself. This suggests that the factors that contribute to a woman's "need" to start smoking may also be at work in affecting the size of the baby, even if the mother-to-be has not yet started to smoke. In this view, that is, smoking is considered an indirect rather than a direct causal factor in low birth weight.

As might be expected, these results are highly controversial. So many researchers have come to the opposite conclusion—that smoking directly contributes to the decreased weight of newborns. The criticisms have been many. One problem that has been raised is that the future smokers—those nonsmokers who took up the habit after pregnancy—were several years younger than the women who smoked during pregnancy. This difference may have affected the results and contributed to the lower birth weights of the babies of the future smokers. Younger women, the future smokers, are more likely to be having a first baby and, in general, firstborns are lighter than babies born to older women who previously have had children. Thus, the critics argue, the lighter babies of the future smokers may reflect the younger age of these women. A second serious issue is that very often the women were asked to recall their smoking habits during pregnancies that occurred a number of years earlier. Such recollections may well be inaccurate. Finally, the critics say, some elements that are known to influence birth weight, such as the sex of the baby and the number of previous pregnancies, were not taken into consideration.

More recent work that has attempted to take into account at least some of these criticisms has not clearly settled the issue of whether the smoker rather than the smoking causes the reduction in birth weight. The present status of this controversy appears to be that the evidence is just too overwhelming to disclaim that smoking has a direct effect on fetal growth. This is not to deny that factors that differentiate smokers from nonsmokers (other than the use or nonuse of cigarettes) may influence the newborn's weight. Rather, the existence of these factors and the extent of their influence on birth weight still remain to be clearly demonstrated and quantified.

At the beginning of this chapter it was pointed out that babies who are small at birth can be categorized in one of two ways. In one instance the baby is born well before the 280-day gestation period is completed. This newborn, called a preterm baby, is small simply because he or she has not had the normal period of time to grow. In the second instance the infants are smaller than average for the length of time that they have been carried, whether this be preterm or fullterm. These babies are called small for dates.

The association of smoking with a lowered average size at birth and an increased frequency of low birth weight infants raises an obvious question. Does the difference between babies born to nonsmokers and smokers represent a reduction in the length of gestation in the latter group, resulting in a preterm infant, or are the babies small for dates? The evidence is clear on this point. Smoking during pregnancy causes a negligible shortening of gestation. Typically, the average difference between smokers and nonsmokers is in the neighborhood of two days. This slight decrease in the length of pregnancy is certainly not sufficient to account for the differences in birth weight that are usually reported. An often quoted figure is that the difference in the duration of pregnancy between smokers and nonsmokers can account for less than 10 percent of the discrepancies in birth weight of infants born to these two groups of women.

The answer to the question of whether the lighter birth weight and increased incidence of low birth weight babies among smoking mothers reflect preterm or small for date infants is quite clear. Smoking increases the probability of having a small for dates infant, that is, an infant whose rate of fetal growth is reduced. This increased probability of a slowing of fetal growth occurs in babies of all gestational ages: fullterm, preterm, and even postterm (several weeks overdue). One comes to this conclusion by comparing the babies of smokers and nonsmokers who were born at different gestational ages. No matter how many weeks less or more than the normal, forty-week gestational period the pregnancy may be, the average birth weight of a baby born to a mother who smoked during pregnancy is likely to be less than the weight of a baby of the same gestational age born to a nonsmoker.

One mechanism by which smoking during pregnancy

may cause a reduced birth weight is via the mother's food intake. This proposition has been criticized for a number of reasons. As mentioned in Chapter 4, many researchers have failed to find evidence that mothers who smoke during pregnancy gain less weight than those who do not smoke, a finding that they argue does not reflect differences in food intake. As also discussed in Chapter 4, among those workers who have found differences in smokers' and nonsmokers' weight gain during pregnancy two interpretations have been put forth. One body of thought is that the woman who smokes has a lowered appetite, lessened food intake, and, consequently, a more slowly growing fetus. The opinion expressed by other researchers is that smoking has a direct effect upon the fetus and retards fetal growth. This slowing of the growth of the unborn baby is then reflected in a diminished weight gain of the mother-to-be.

The most recent evidence does not support the idea that reduced appetite retards the growth of the fetus in smoking women. Two different lines of evidence converge to lead to this conclusion. The first involves work that demonstrated that full term, low birth weight babies can be of two general appearances. One group of infants is described as being long and thin, whereas the others have short body lengths for their gestational dates.

Babies born to mothers who suffer from malnutrition during pregnancy are often described in the scientific literature as long and thin. Therefore, if a lessening of appetite during pregnancy results in a diminution of food intake so that the fetus's growth is reduced because of nutritional deprivation, the newborn should be long and thin. In fact, however, small for dates babies born to smoking mothers are symmetrically small. That is, everything about them is small: body length, head circumference, and weight. This suggests that the fetal growth retardation associated with smoking is the result not of malnutrition brought about by decreased food intake but rather of some other factor.

There is a second line of research indicating that maternal weight gain and the effects of smoking on birth weight are independent. Smokers and nonsmokers who gained the same amount of weight during pregnancy were compared. The comparisons involved women who gained as little as five pounds right up to women who gained over forty pounds. Within any particular level of maternal weight gain, in comparing smokers and nonsmokers, it was found that the more the mother-to-be smoked the greater the likelihood that the infant would be a low birth baby. The consistency of this difference between smokers and nonsmokers across the wide range of maternal weight gains suggests that smoking rather than a reduction in maternal nutrition has a direct effect on the growth of the unborn baby.

As discussed in Chapter 5, the placenta is the communicating link between the mother and the unborn child. As such it is quite logical and natural to examine this structure in order to see whether it can shed some light on the mechanisms that result in the increased frequency of small for dates babies born to smoking mothers. Several studies were undertaken to investigate how smoking may affect the placenta. The general finding was that the weight of this structure is either unaffected or affected only slightly by smoking. Light smokers were found to have placentas that were similar to or slightly lighter than those of nonsmokers whereas heavy smokers had placentas that weighed slightly more than those of nonsmokers. However, no matter what level of smoking was considered, most workers found that if the placental weight were considered as a fraction of the birth weight of the baby, the resulting placental ratio was higher among smoking than among nonsmoking mothers. This increased placental ratio comes about because there is essentially little difference between smokers and nonsmokers with respect to placental weight, whereas there usually is a dose related reduction in birth weight. Thus, the ratio of placental weight to birth weight increases as the amount of smoking of the mother-to-be increases.

Does this higher placental ratio have any significance with respect to a central issue of this chapter—smoking and small for dates infants? The answer is definitely yes. Besides the case of the mother-to-be who smokes, two other situations are associated with increased placental ratios. One such instance occurs when pregnancy occurs at high altitudes and the other occurs when the pregnant woman is anemic. In both of these cases the availability of oxygen for the fetus is reduced. It has been proposed that the enlargement of the placenta relative to the size of the fetus is a physiological response to the decreased amount of oxygen carried by the mother. The increased placental ratio serves to increase the opportunity of transfering oxygen from mother to fetus.

As discussed in Chapter 2, the smoking mother-to-be has a decreased ability to carry oxygen as the hemoglobin in her blood, which normally carries oxygen, is now carrying considerable amounts of carbon monoxide. Thus, as in other cases in which the amount of oxygen available for the fetus is reduced, the higher placental ratio may be a protective mechanism serving to increase the opportunity for oxygen transfer to take place.

This research with placental ratios provides indirect evidence that the oxygen available to the fetus of smoking mothers is less than that available to the unborn of nonsmokers. This finding, coupled with the direct evidence of reduced oxygen in the blood of smoking mothers, has led most workers to conclude that the major contributing factor to the birth weight differences between the babies of smokers and nonsmokers is related to insufficient oxygen. Babies born at high altitudes also have a reduced birth weight. This is presumably linked to the shortage of oxygen available, at such altitudes, to the fetus. The similar effect noted among maternal smokers supports the interpretation that oxygen deficiency accounts for reduced weight among the babies of these women. Obviously, the increased placental ratio found both in smoking mothers and in women at high altitudes is not a sufficient physiological adjustment to overcome oxygen deficiency.

Cigarettes smoked during pregnancy can affect the oxygen needed for the growth of the fetus in at least two ways. The nicotine contained in cigarettes constricts all blood vessels, including those passing through the placenta. This narrowing restricts the quantity of blood and its load of oxygen available to the unborn baby. Smoking also reduces oxygen availability because of the carbon monoxide inhaled in the cigarette smoke. As we have seen, carbon monoxide combines with the blood's hemoglobin to form carboxyhemoglobin in both the mother and the fetus; therefore, the blood's oxygen-carrying capacity in both is reduced.

As with all living organisms, in order for the fetus to grow normally, an adequate, constant supply of oxygen is needed. The decrease in oxygen available to the developing fetus of a smoking mother is thought to be of a magnitude sufficient to retard growth. It is presumed that the tissues of the fetus simply cannot grow to the same extent that they would have had the quantity of oxygen not been reduced by cigarette smoking.

In summary, the evidence that smoking has a direct effect upon the birth weight of an infant is very strong. The average lighter weight (by eight ounces) of babies born to mothers who smoke, the doubled likelihood of a smoker's having a low birth weight baby, the dose response relationship between smoking and birth weight, and the fact that the birth weights of siblings shift with the changing smoking habits of their mother all lead to the same conclusion—a cause and effect association between cigarettes and lowered birth weight. The most likely major mechanism by which smoking affects birth weight is its reduction of the supply of oxygen available to the developing fetus. If fetal growth retardation is in fact caused by oxygen deficiency, the question of whether this result has consequences for the baby other than lowered birth weight is of considerable importance. This issue will be discussed in Chapters 8 and 10.

chapter eight
The Newborn

Although it might be thought that the newborn is entirely a product of what he or she has inherited genetically from the parents, the overwhelming evidence is that this assumption is not valid. For, in addition to the genes, environmental factors influence the growing fetus, their effects manifest in the physiological and behavioral responses of the infant at birth. As we discussed in previous chapters, the mother's general health and the physical and chemical factors transmitted through her are instrumental in fetal development. There is little question that these intrauterine influences play an important role in the intellectual and emotional development of the human infant.

Because of its potential lifelong impact the newborn's physical and psychological state should be assessed at the earliest possible age. The need for this early evaluation lies in the fact that the sooner any physiological or behavioral diagnoses of abnormalities are made, the greater the likelihood that these dysfunctions can be treated successfully. Such identification is not difficult when the abnormality is severe but subtle impairments are a different matter. They require very sensitive techniques that have been developed only recently.

At birth, the baby's world changes in an abrupt, dramatic fashion. From the relatively insulated mother's body the infant is now exposed directly to a wide range of environmental influences. The baby is suddenly required to rely on his or her own coping mechanisms. At a physiological level, the survival of the newborn infant at birth depends primarily upon the immediate expansion of the lungs and the establishment of an exchange of gases, mainly oxygen and carbon dioxide. Normally the baby begins to breathe almost immediately after birth and cries soon afterward. This crying indicates that active respiration has been established and that important modifications in the circulatory system have taken place as the infant adapts to life outside the uterus. The normal newborn will breathe well within one minute of birth and should cry shortly thereafter.

It has been shown that in the fetus rhythmic movements of the wall of the chest and the diaphragm occur beginning in the second trimester of pregnancy. There is, of course, no air to breathe but in response to these respiratory movements, amniotic fluid flows into and out of the passages of the respiratory tract. It is thought that the breathing activity that takes place after birth is a continuation of intrauterine respiration.

These prenatal movements occur thoughout the greater part of pregnancy, increasing as the end of the period of gestation is neared, with the expansions and relaxations taking place at a rate of around thirty per minute. Such movements are quite complex, involving a large number of muscles moving in a precise sequence, and this coordination requires direction from parts of the brain. By studying the proportion of time that the fetus makes breathing movements and the patterns of these movements, information about the maturation and functioning of the nervous system can be obtained.

The smoking of cigarettes by the mother-to-be has a marked effect on fetal breathing movements. If a pregnant woman smokes as few as two consecutive cigarettes there is a marked reduction in the overall amount of time that her fetus spends making breathing movements. One would think that the major contributing factor to this decrease would have to do with the production of carbon monoxide and its interference with oxygen availability for the fetus. Surprisingly, this does not appear to be the case. Rather, the culprit seems to be nicotine. This was shown in a study in which two types of cigarettes were smoked by pregnant women. Some of the cigarettes were the usual kind, but the others were made from material that did not contain any nicotine. Both forms of cigarettes produced carbon monoxide, but only the ones containing nicotine markedly reduced the breathing movements of the fetus.

If indeed these reduced movements are a reflection of the functioning of parts of the fetal brain, the results suggest that the nicotine passing through the placenta can depress certain activities of the nervous system. A critical question is whether such alterations are evident at and immediately after birth.

At the time of delivery the newborn is examined to assess its general status. The color of the baby's skin is a measure of the circulation. With the onset of respiration the skin changes color, from a dusky to a ruddy tone. The first breath is normally taken within seconds of birth and the first cry within half a minute. Immediate urination is a good sign that the baby's "plumbing" is in order.

A system of evaluating the condition of the newborn infant on the basis of a numerical score was worked out by Virginia Apgar in 1952. Five parameters—heart rate, respiratory effort, muscular tone, reflex responses, and color—are appraised at one and at five minutes after birth. Each of these factors is assigned zero, one, or two points, and these scores are added together. Most babies are normal and receive seven to ten total points. A score of four to six indicates the presence of mild to moderate asphyxia (insufficient breathing). When the Apgar score is zero, one, or two, the infant is severely depressed and in danger.

The relationship between smoking and the Apgar score has been considered in a number of investigations. Two approaches to this question can be taken. One may try to deter-

Table 8-1
The Apgar Score

Sign	0 points	1 point	2 points
Heart rate	absent	under 100	over 100
Respiratory effort	absent	slow, irregular	good, crying
Muscle tone	limp	flexion of extremities	active motion
Reflex—response to stimulation of the nostril	no response	grimace	cough or sneeze
Color	blue-white	body pink, extremities blue	completely pink

mine whether infants born to smokers are more likely than babies born to nonsmoking mothers to fall into the low and potentially dangerous Apgar scoring categories. An alternative approach is to measure the average Apgar scores of infants from the two groups of mothers noting whether there are any consistent differences.

Both of these approaches give essentially the same result. It does not appear that maternal smoking increases the likelihood of the newborn's having a score of less than four on the Apgar scale. Nor does smoking during pregnancy result consistently in a reduction of the average Apgar value. Although there has been one report of slightly lowered Apgar scores among babies born to smoking mothers, several other studies have failed to find any such reduction. Even in the single investigation that did associate lower Apgar scores with maternal smoking, the extent of the reduction was so small that it had no clinical significance.

The Apgar score is a valuable method of assessing the newborn's capacity to respond to the stress of labor, delivery, and adjustment to a new environment. However, this evaluative tool is really only a measure of the capacity of the infant to cope with its new status in the first five minutes of life. It does not give a good indication of how the baby will do afterward. In addition, the Apgar score is a subjective assessment and as such is prone to considerable variation from one observer to another. In the 1970s techniques for assessing the very young infant have mushroomed in number in an attempt to find ways to identify physical and psychological characteristics that are predictive of the baby's future performance.

Most of these newer tests are directed at relatively complex behavior. It is somewhat surprising to think that an infant of only a few days of age can exhibit behavior that can be termed complex and that such behavior can be measured. But there is little doubt that this is the case.

Immediately after birth the newborn baby is active. He or she does not lie quietly but moves around. This movement, despite what it might look like superficially, is not random. The baby responds to stimulation. He or she will turn his or her head to the side from which a voice is coming and seems to be searching for the face of the speaker. The normal baby is capable of integrating visual, auditory, and motor behavior in response to human stimuli. The capacities of the newborn in the areas of vision, hearing, smell, taste, sensitivity to touch, and smoking can be examined and evaluated.

Even during the first few days of life, if any of the sensory systems and their connections with the nervous system are not functioning normally there is likely to be an interference with the newborn's capacity to process the wealth of information to which he or she is being exposed. Sensory deficits at a very young age can also interfere with some of the earliest learning that the infant does—namely, the development of adaptive responses to new stimuli. At a more general level, if the baby is very irritable and cannot be consoled, his or her ability to take in, cope with, and adapt to the surrounding environment is bound to be reduced. Continuous irritability is also likely to have a negative effect upon the reaction of the mother and father, and a vicious circle of anxiety and frustration may result.

Many of the recently developed tests are designed to assess the infant's capacity to interact with the environment by noting not only the newborn's sensory capabilities but also certain nonsensory aspects of behavior. The latter include observations of how long the infant stays in various states of arousal, including attentiveness, apathy, irritability, and hyperexcitability, and when these periods occur. Each one of these states represents particular levels of nervous system activity.

Perhaps because these infant developmental assessment techniques are so new, very few reports in the research literature have compared the babies of smokers and non-smokers utilizing these procedures. A particular innovative approach that has been used, however, is the Brazelton Neonatal Assessment Scale, first described in 1973 and now used in over two hundred research centers.

This is one of the very few tests that looks at the effects of maternal smoking upon the state of the baby's nervous system and his or her capacity to interact with the environment. For this reason, and because the testing procedures are so interesting in their own right, it is worthwhile to go into the techniques in a little detail.

The first part of the testing procedure involves the examination of the newborn's capacity to ignore stimuli to which he or she does not wish to pay attention or respond. Such absence of responding is tested in several ways. For example, a fairly loud bell is shaken near the baby's ear when the infant is in a drowsy state. Typically the infant's reaction is to startle, with both arms and legs moving vigorously, eyes blinking open, and breathing rate increased. If the noise is repeated at approximately five-second intervals, most babies will continue to show these startles after each of the first two or three shakes of the bell. But typically on the subsequent presentations of the noisy bell a remarkable thing occurs. The newborn's startle reduces in vigor and by the eighth or ninth ring of the bell many infants seem not to respond at all and, in fact, go back to their drowsy, semi-sleeping state. This shutdown in responding is not limited to auditory stimuli. A similar sequence of events occurs when a light is flashed repeatedly into the baby's eyes.

The capacity to shut out unwanted, repetitive stimuli and to control startle responses is a useful adaptive ability for the newborn to have. Not only does it help the baby cope with the new, bright, noisy environment by neutralizing the disturbing nature of the many stimuli, but the diminution of the startle response helps conserve the relatively small amount of energy that the infant has. A further dramatic example of the rapid ability of the normal newborn to minimize unnecessary activity is seen in the Brazelton test when the baby's foot is lightly pricked with a pin. Initially a startle will result, both feet will be withdrawn, and fussing and thrashing behavior will follow. If the pinpricks are repeated at regular intervals most babies will stop most of their vigorous reactions, the only response being a pushing away with one foot. As in the case of the noise and the light, the newborn's response to the repeated unpleasant stimulus diminishes rapidly so that eventually only the essential components remain, thereby minimizing the amount of energy used.

This ability of the newborn to control responses to the environment is a complex process and is felt to reflect a maturing, healthy nervous system. When an infant has difficulty in decreasing and limiting responses to the multitude of continuous stimuli to which he or she is inevitably exposed, this *may* be a symptom of a subtle abnormality of the nervous system. For example, the baby may react to all stimuli with vigorous startle responses. Not only is the baby overwhelmed with the input but also, quite naturally, the infant becomes exhausted. Such babies tend to spend a lot of time sleeping and crying. Perhaps it is more than coincidental that both of these types of behavior result in shutting out stimuli from the new environment.

Besides testing the ability of the baby to shut out unwanted stimuli, the Brazelton technique examines the infant's capacity to choose what he or she wants to respond to. For example, the newborn infant will often turn toward a soft human voice, quiet down, and appear to look around as if searching for the source of the sound. When the baby catches sight of the adult's face, particularly the eyes, the newborn will often focus on the face for a few minutes. There is no question that the infant can see. Moreover, if the source of the voice continues to talk softly and slowly moves his or her head, the newborn will typically follow the face while reducing those leg and arm movements that may interfere with this tracking. During the Brazelton examination the newborn's ability to turn the head and eyes in different directions in order to locate the source of the voice and the degree to which the eyes follow a slowly moving face are noted. Similar tests are also carried out using an inanimate object such as a ball. Once the ball is visually picked up by the baby, the extent of tracking is observed.

A variety of reflexive behaviors are also tested during the Brazelton examination. The range of reflexes that the newborn is capable of is surprising. For example, a walking reflex can be elicited by holding the newborn in an upright position with the feet on a hard surface and leaning the baby forward. A Moro reflex occurs when the infant experiences a sudden movement. It consists of an initial startle response, during which the baby throws out the arms, followed by a bringing back of the arms together as if to hold on to anyone close by. By gently stroking the side of the mouth two reflexes can be set off. The baby will turn the mouth and often the tongue toward the stroking stimulus, and sucking movements of the mouth frequently will occur.

The strength and the way in which the reflexes express themselves are useful indicators of the status of the nervous system. Abnormalities of the nervous system may prevent the reflexes from being performed in a normal, smooth way or may result in an undue amount of tremors.

Throughout the testing period general characteristics of the baby are noted. These include muscular strength, irritability, alertness, the amount of tremors, the extent of crying, and the ease with which the baby can be consoled. As can be seen, the Brazelton Neonatal Assessment Scale considers the newborn infant as anything but a passive receiver of information. This testing procedure, which takes about thirty minutes to administer, is a sensitive assessment for a wide range of behaviors that reflect nervous system functioning.

In 1978 the Brazelton scale was used to compare the babies of mothers who smoked during pregnancy and those whose mothers did not smoke. The two groups of mothers were quite similar, however, with regard to other factors that may affect the newborn's behavior. These factors included the age of the woman, her social class, the number of previous births, the length of labor, and medication given during labor.

The babies were tested between four and six days of age. Two basic differences were noted: one existed in responsiveness and disposition and the other in a specific sensory system. In contrast to the infants born to nonsmoking women, the babies of mothers who smoked tended to be more irritable, had less ability to control their own behavior, and displayed a general lack of interest. In addition to these general differences in overall behavior, hearing in the babies of the maternal smokers appeared to be impaired or reduced. In the tests that examine the infant's responsiveness to both the human voice and the bell, the infants born to smokers were less responsive.

In an investigation currently under way in our research facilities in hospitals in Ottawa, we are administering the Brazelton test to infants between two and five days of age born to smoking and nonsmoking mothers. As in the study just described, the women in the two groups are similar with respect to age, social class, previous births, and medication during labor. We also have taken into account the drinking habits of the women because several investigators have shown that alcohol consumed regularly during pregnancy can affect the newborn's performance on the Brazelton examination.

Our results are strikingly similar to those of the previous study. We are finding that the babies born to maternal smokers do not respond to sound to the same degree as do the infants of nonsmokers. Also, as in the earlier work, there is greater irritability among the babies of the smoking women.

The dispositional and auditory changes associated with maternal smoking are coupled with some additional effects in the newborns of the smoking mothers. As we described earlier, parts of the Brazelton Neonatal Assessment Scale are designed specifically to examine the degree to which a baby can shut out unwanted stimuli. In our work we have found that the infants of maternal smokers are consistently less able to diminish or to cease totally their response to repetitive visual or auditory stimuli. The differences between the two groups of babies are marked. Infants in the nonsmoking group stop giving any pronounced response after four or five presentations of either the light or the sound. On the other hand, babies born to smokers do not reduce significantly their level of startle and bodily movement even after nine or ten presentations of a stimulus.

Another difference in the babies we have examined relates to a behavior that occurs repeatedly throughout the entire testing period. We have found that infants born to smoking mothers consistently display many more tremors in their arms and legs compared to the babies of nonsmokers. These tremors occur both when the infants are crying and when they are not.

These two studies represent the current level of information regarding the effect of maternal smoking upon the newborn's behavior. The fact that the number of studies is so small makes it impossible to come to any definitive conclusion at this time. However, as both investigations have had common findings associated with smoking during pregnancy, some tentative statements can be made.

The increase in irritability and in other behaviors indicative of discomfort that has been seen among many of the babies of maternal smokers may be related to the phenomenon of nicotine withdrawal. When adults who have been regular smokers give up cigarettes their bodies protest. The symptoms are well known to those who have gone this route. In addition to the craving for a cigarette, there is irritability, restlessness, sleep disturbance, headaches, and impaired concentration. These symptoms occur typically within a matter of hours after the last cigarette and may persist for months.

The causes underlying these withdrawal pangs have not been specifically identified, but the evidence suggests that both the interruption of the habitual act of smoking and the decrease of nicotine in the body contribute to the symptoms. It is the latter of these two that is important in our discussion.

It is generally accepted that regular smokers adjust the number of cigarettes smoked and the rate and degree of inhalation in order to produce a relatively stable level of nicotine in the circulatory system. To demonstrate this fact, investigators gave heavy smokers their regular brand of cigarettes with either more or less nicotine than normal. When the switch from the regular cigarettes to cigarettes with the higher nicotine content occurred, the smokers reduced considerably the number of cigarettes they lit up, and the nicotine values in their blood remained almost identical to the values found when they smoked their own brand. In other words, without realizing it the smokers were smoking only enough cigarettes containing the large amount of nicotine to maintain those levels of nicotine in the body to which they were accustomed. When the smokers were given the cigarettes with a low content of nicotine the reverse occurred, that is, more cigarettes were smoked. Presumably, this increase was also an attempt to keep the nicotine in the blood at the usual level.

When a regular smoker stops the cigarette habit the nicotine level in the blood falls and the symptoms described earlier occur. The type and the extent of withdrawal signs vary markedly among individuals. This difference occurs not only because the particular nicotine level in the blood contributes to the psychological and physiological disturbances, but also because such factors as personality and the ways in which stress is handled by the individual affect the expression of the withdrawal symptoms.

During pregnancy, as we discussed in previous chapters, some of the nicotine that the mother inhales through her cigarettes passes through the placenta and comes into contact with the developing fetus. Thus, if the mother is a regular smoker the unborn baby's circulatory system will be carrying nicotine.

At birth, the baby is suddenly removed from the source of nicotine. If, as appears reasonable to assume, the infant had adjusted during gestation to the nicotine level in his or her blood, the sudden lack of the substance at birth would have consequences parallel to the withdrawal symptoms experienced by adults. The notion of nicotine withdrawal in the newborn is consistent with what we know happens with other drugs upon which a dependency is developed by the pregnant woman. On a much more severe scale, babies born to narcotics users go through several days of marked withdrawal symptoms. For example, infants whose mothers used heroin during pregnancy display a large amount of irritability, tremors, shrill, high-pitched crying, poor feeding, vomiting, and diarrhea typically for about a week.

As we have seen in the two studies concerned with maternal smokers' babies during the first few days of life, such infants tend to display more crying, tremors, and irritability than babies born to nonsmokers. These behaviors are the only way by which the infant can express discomfort. Underlying the baby's distress may be the physical disturbances associated with the withdrawal of nicotine.

The observation was made in both studies that hearing may be affected among the newborns of smoking mothers. Although at first glance it would appear reasonable to attribute the effect to maternal smoking, other factors may also be playing a role. For example, in Chapter 7 we discussed the possible role in lowered birth weight of the smoker herself rather than the act of smoking. A similar possibility exists in the present situation. That is, perhaps there is a difference between smokers and nonsmokers other than their use or nonuse of cigarettes that may influence the development of the auditory system of the fetus.

In spite of this necessary caution in attributing a cause and effect relationship between smoking during pregnancy and hearing defects in the newborn, some evidence points to a direct link.

In earlier chapters we discussed how smoking during pregnancy causes an increase in carbon monoxide in the body. We indicated how this in turn decreases the oxygen-carrying capacity of the blood, as carboxyhemogloblin forms in the mother-to-be and in the fetus. We also discussed how smoking decreases the amount of blood flowing through the uterus and placenta by decreasing the diameter of the blood vessels.

In adults carboxyhemoglobin (even at low levels) has been shown to affect hearing and a reduced blood flow following smoking has been suggested as a major cause of hearing loss.

If carboxyhemoglobin and reduced blood flow affect the adult's hearing, it is probable that they influence the development of parts of the ear in the fetus. If so, the consequence would likely be a deficiency in hearing as noted in two studies. It must be emphasized that in neither study were babies found to be deaf; rather, maternal smoking was associated with subtle impairments of the newborn's hearing.

The long-term consequences of such a deficit remain to be determined. For example, would such an impairment delay slightly the beginning of verbal communication? How about performance at school?

As mentioned earlier in this chapter, the ability of the newborn to tune out repeated, unimportant stimuli is considered by some workers to be one indication of a healthy, well-functioning nervous system. The finding that maternal smoking appears to be associated with the infant's inability to reduce the amount of responding as the same stimulus is presented over and over may be a clue that smoking is having some subtle effect upon the nervous system. The apparent association between smoking during pregnancy and the presence of more than the usual amount of tremors in the newborn also may be indicative of the effects of smoking upon the nervous system of the fetus.

If smoking during pregnancy does have subtle effect upon the nervous system of the unborn baby, the most likely mechanism by which it is causing damage is through the increased level of carboxyhemoglobin and the related decrease in oxygen available to the fetus.

About a century ago coal miners took cages containing canaries down into the shafts with them. They did not take the birds along because of their singing ability. Rather, the birds accompanied the miners because canaries are far more sensitive than people to the dangerous carbon monoxide gas that frequently is present in mines. When the birds were overcome by the gas and fell off their perches, the men were forewarned of danger well before they themselves could detect it. It has been argued that the fetus in the mother is analogous to the canaries in that the unborn baby is extremely sensitive to carbon monoxide and the oxygen deficiency it causes.

One of the most unfortunate aspects of this sensitivity is

that the effects of the oxygen depletion are not seen until after the damage may have been done: at birth, months later, or even years later. The lack of response diminution and the tremors may be early signs of the effects on the sensitive fetus of carbon monoxide. In Chapter 10 we will discuss whether there are indications that oxygen reduction in the fetus has consequences that go beyond the first few days of life.

chapter nine
Breast Milk and Nursing

Each month, under the influence of the hormones estrogen and progesterone, produced in the ovaries, the breasts undergo preparation for pregnancy. If conception does not take place, the levels of the hormones drop, menstruation follows, and the breasts return to the prehormonal state. When conception does occur, the production of hormones increases and the development of the breasts proceeds in preparation for lactation.

Three factors play an important role in both the initiation and the maintenance of nursing: the anatomical structure of the breasts, the production of milk, and the ejection of milk from the interior of the breast to the nipple. A brief description of each component will help make it easier to understand how smoking may interact with breastfeeding.

Each breast is made up of from fifteen to twenty sections known as lobes, which are separated from each other by varying amounts of fat. The size and shape of the breasts depend mainly on the content of fat but, as most women know, size does not bear on whether or not a mother will be successful at nursing. Each of the many lobes of the breast is subdivided into lobules and each of these contains a large number of small secreting glands, the active producers of milk. Each lobule has a small duct that joins with other ducts coming from other lobules; together the small ducts form a single larger duct that drains a lobe. These larger ducts, like branches on a tree close to the trunk, come together in the area of the nipple, where they open on the surface. Around the nipple is a circular, darkened area called the areola. The surface of the areola is somewhat rough because just below the skin in this area are small glands that lubricate the nipple. Muscles in the areola function to make the nipple stiffen so that the nursing baby can get a better grasp with its mouth while sucking.

In the pregnant woman several changes occur that make the production of milk possible. The small ducts and the lobules in the breasts increase in number and the placenta secretes hormones in large quantities that stimulate the growth of the breasts. In ordinary circumstances women are not capable of producing milk without the preparation of the breasts that is undergone during pregnancy; however, the ability of non-expectant women to successfully nurse is a historical fact. There are two ways that this comes about and in both cases it is a matter of essentially fooling the body into thinking that there is a need for the milk. The more commonly reported procedure is for the woman to continue to empty her breasts long after her infant has weaned. The body interprets this stimulation as a continuing need of a hungry baby and persists in the manufacture and excretion of milk. A less common means of stimulating lactation has been reported by women who responded to vigorous suckling of other women's infants or adopted babies with increased growth of the breasts and the production of milk.

For approximately two to six days after birth the breasts do not contain real milk, but a small amount of a thick, yellowish liquid called colostrum can be expressed from the nipples. Colostrum contains more protein, less sugar, and much less fat than milk. The shift to milk occurs roughly two to six days after birth and usually by the end of the first week the secretion of milk is well established. With first babies, however, the establishment of lactation may take several weeks longer.

One of the chief values of colostrum and breast milk is

that they both contain antibodies that protect the newborn against infection. The type and number of antibodies reaching the baby depend on the mother's level of immunity resulting either from artificial immunization or from previous infection. Several studies have shown that the incidence of infection is lower among babies who are breastfed.

The nutritional aspects of breast milk and how they are tied to the young baby's needs are described later in this chapter. However, a few general comments can be made at this time. Over a hundred constituents have been identified in breast milk but the essential nutritional components are a mixture of protein, sugar, salts, vitamins, minerals, and a variety of fatty compounds. The percentages of these compounds differ from individual to individual and even within a particular woman the composition of the milk changes not only from day to day but also during any given day. In terms of nutritional content the milk is relatively unaffected by the state of nutrition of the mother. Even during famines women often manage to feed their babies relatively well.

The quantity, as opposed to the quality, of milk depends to a considerable degree on the amount of fluid ingested by the mother. In addition, it is estimated that about one thousand calories per day are required to produce the energy used in the secretion of the milk so that a mother's intake of food ought to reflect this new demand.

The birth of a baby sets off a series of complicated hormonal interactions in the mother that lead to the production of milk by the glands of the breasts. Occasionally on the second day after delivery and nearly always by the third or fourth day, the breasts become larger, firmer, and sometimes somewhat painful. This is a sign that secretion of milk has begun.

There are two parts to the process of lactation. In the first phase, that of secretion, milk is produced by and stored in the numerous mammary glands of the breast. The amount of milk produced is controlled to a large degree by a hor-

91

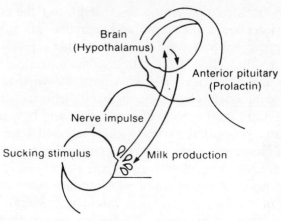

Figure 9-1. The basic features of milk production. The sucking of the baby sends nerve impulses to the hypothalamus in the brain. The hypothalamus stimulates the anterior pituitary gland to release prolactin, which promotes milk production in the mammary glands.

mone called prolactin. As Figure 9–1 illustrates, this hormone is secreted by a gland at the base of the brain, the anterior pituitary, in response to messages from the hypothalamus in the brain. The prolactin is carried in the bloodstream to the breast, where it acts on the milk producing cells. The more prolactin secreted by the anterior pituitary, the more milk secreted in the mammary glands. In order for milk production to be maintained, hormones from the anterior pituitary gland must continue to be released. This release comes about in response to stimulation of the nipple. If sucking by the infant is stopped, the secretion of the necessary hormones by the pituitary gland into the bloodstream ceases and usually milk production virtually stops within a few days.

In order for the milk to be made available to the infant it has to be ejected from the mammary glands into the large ducts that lead to the nipples. This is the second step in the

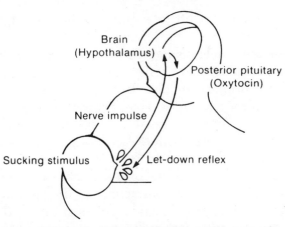

Figure. 9-2. The basic features of milk ejection, or the letdown reflex. The sucking of the baby sends nerve impulses to the hypothalamus in the brain. The hypothalamus stimulates the posterior pituitary gland to release oxytocin, which causes the contraction of musclelike cells around the milk producing glands. This causes the milk to be ejected through the ducts to the nipple, where it becomes available to the nursing baby.

process of lactation. Again, the baby plays a critical role in milk ejection, or the let-down reflex, as Figure 9-2 shows. Sucking on the nipple triggers impulses to the brain, which in turn relays a stimulus to the posterior pituitary gland. This gland releases the hormone oxytocin into the bloodstream, which carries it to the breasts. Oxytocin acts on musclelike cells that surround the milk producing cells. These muscle cells contract when oxytocin reaches them and squeezes the milk from the site of manufacture into the duct system; from when the nursing baby can readily suckle.

The let-down reflex is quite sensitive to small differences in oxytocin levels in the blood. Such levels are influenced by emotional and psychological disturbances. Anxiety can retard the let-down reflex and confidence can enhance it. For example, milk ejection can be inhibited by embarrassment or stress and can be set off in a nursing mother by the mere thought of her baby or the infant's cry.

These are numerous indications to the nursing mother that a successful let-down reflex has occurred. She may experience the dripping of milk from the breasts after (and sometimes even before) the baby starts to nurse, the milk being expelled from the breast opposite to the one being nursed. Also associated with the let-down reflex are cramps of the uterus while nursing in the first few days after birth. These occur because the same oxytocin that causes the milk to be released also causes contractions of the uterus.

Thus, for both processes involved in lactation, the production and the release of milk, sucking stimulation is the key initiator. This helps explain how, as described earlier, women are able to produce milk though they have not been pregnant.

Under normal circumstances the baby ought to be put to the breast as soon as possible but not later than twelve hours after birth both to stimulate the breasts and to obtain the very valuable pre-milk colostrum. Some women, due to particular circumstances, cannot nurse their babies. Others simply do not care to nurse. To such the following advantages of breast over artificial milk should be pointed out: (1) psychological—the baby gets a sense of security and acceptance from and by the person in all the world most important to him or her—a not negligible matter in this increasingly neurotic age; (2) there is no milk like breast milk; and (3) breast milk is always handy, always warm, and always sterile.

Many, if not all, products ingested by the mother are excreted in the milk in some form. Fortunately the amount is small, and the vast majority have clinically insignificant effects on the infant. Still, care must be exercised to make certain that the mother is not taking any drug that could be injurious to the baby.

Small amounts of alcohol do not affect the production

of milk, but large quantities reduce the milk ejecting response. Cathartics may cause the infant to have colic, abdominal pain, and diarrhea. Opium and its derivatives, atropine, salicylates, iodides, bromides, quinine, lead, and mercury are excreted into the milk and may harm the baby. Nicotine from cigarettes is transmitted in breast milk. However, the evidence regarding the harmful effects on the breastfeeding infant of maternal smoking is scanty, contradictory, and inconclusive. Before going over the data that are available, it is useful to discuss briefly why the very young baby has particular nutritional demands.

The first year of life, more than any other period, is a time of rapid growth and development. Maturation of the body and the nervous system is dependent upon an appropriate intake of calories and nutrients.

During the first twelve months the nutritional needs of the infant differ considerably from those of a child or an adult. There are three general reasons for this. First, the makeup of the infant's body is different; second, the physical activity, particularly during the first four months, is minimal; and third, the infant's growth rate is more rapid at this time than during any subsequent period.

In the first four months of postnatal life between a quarter and a third of the energy taken in by the infant is used up in the growing process. During this 120-day period the baby may double his or her birth weight and usually spends a lot of time sleeping. The energy needs of the low birth weight infant are often higher during this period than those of a heavier baby in order to catch up.

Between four months and a year there is a shift in the utilization of nourishment. Now only about 10 percent of the food is needed for growth while a greater proportion is used to provide the energy for the marked increase in activity that occurs during this period.

At birth the organs (for example, brain, liver, gut, heart, and kidney) make up about 15 percent of the total body weight; the muscle, 25 percent; fat, 12 percent; and bone and connective tissue, 15 percent. The remainder of the body weight is made up of the fluids that surround all the tissues. As the baby gets older different components grow at different rates. The organs and muscles increase in mass at the same rate as the total body weight but not so the other components. The fluid bathing the tissues increases at a slower rate and fat at a faster rate.

By the end of twelve months the average baby weighs three times its birth weight, with the various organs and muscles comprising the same percentage as they did at birth. However, the percentage of fluids surrounding the tissues is down from the 33 percent at birth to 25 percent whereas the percentage of fat has almost doubled. After the first year the organs slow down their growth while the muscles, bones, and fat increase their mass at a faster rate.

The sequence of events in normal overall growth and the changes in the relative size of the different parts of the body require a special nutritional intake. Although here is not the place to detail the evidence, researchers agree that human milk, particularly during the first few months of life, is superior to all other forms of food. The superiority of breast milk lies in the fact that its nutritional content is matched to the infant's nutritional needs during the first year of life. In addition, as mentioned earlier in this chapter, breast milk contains protective immunological substances that are particularly important during the first few weeks. Thus, as long as there is a sufficient quantity of human milk, nursing appears to be the optimal way of meeting the infant's nutritional requirements.

In the 1970s there was an increase in the number of women who breastfed. It has been estimated that twice as many women nurse their babies immediately after birth now as did twenty years ago. However, over half of these women stop breastfeeding within a few months. Why?

Certainly one important factor is that a significant number of mothers are in the work force and find it inconvenient to nurse the infant and work at the same time. In other instances, nursing is stopped because of physiological reasons, including an inadequate volume of milk.

In view of the apparent advantages of breastfeeding and the renewed interest in nursing, the question of the possible interaction between smoking and lactation is of concern to a large number of women. In a book describing the health care of the fetus and the newborn it was suggested that mothers who worked in tobacco factories ought to be aware of the possibility of transmitting some ill effects of tobacco to their babies through nursing. This warning appeared in a medical text written at the turn of this century. In the years since that warning, many issues regarding breastfeeding and cigarette smoking have been raised but, unfortunately, few clear answers have been obtained.

Two facts are generally agreed upon. If the woman who is breastfeeding is a regular smoker, some of the nicotine from the cigarettes will be found in her milk. And, as one might expect, the more the mother smokes the more nicotine in the milk. But these facts raise more questions than they answer. For example, the constituents of milk and the proportions of these constituents vary from the beginning to the end of a feeding. It is not known whether nicotine is found in greater concentrations at any one particular time during the feeding or whether the nicotine content of the milk is essentially the same throughout a nursing session. It is also not established whether the amount of nicotine that the nursing baby receives from breast milk has any effect on the baby. There have been reports of babies displaying various clinical signs of mild nicotine poisoning when they were being nursed by women who smoked. These symptoms—including restlessness, vomiting, loose stools, and increased heart rate—were reported to lessen and then to disappear as the breastfeeding mothers stopped smoking. On the other hand, there have been as many reports of no ill effects from nicotine in suckling babies of smoking mothers.

To date all work has been directed at whether there are

immediate visible effects of the nicotine upon the infants. Obviously, even this relatively straightforward question cannot be answered until more information is gathered. The equally if not more important issue of whether there are more subtle, longer term effects of nicotine in breast milk has not received any thorough investigation. What is the effect on the baby of the combination of involuntary smoking (see Chapter 2) and the nicotine in the milk? Is there a cumulative effect? These are problems that remain to be investigated.

One aspect of smoking and nursing that has received some attention is the question of whether breastfeeding is jeoparized by the mother's cigarette habit. In one study, among women questioned a few days after giving birth, the percentage of smokers among nursing mothers was approximately a third less than that among bottle feeding women. Several interpretations are possible for such a finding. One is that women who breastfeed may be somewhat more health conscious than those who do not and thus less likely to smoke. Or, smoking might interfere with lactation itself and reduce the supply of milk produced so that not enough is available for the baby.

Several physicians have made the general observation that the incidence of an inadequate quantity of breast milk appears higher among smokers than among nonsmokers. Unfortunately, no large surveys of carefully matched smokers and nonsmokers have specifically examined smoking habits and nursing difficulties.

One interesting study supportive of the idea that smoking may interfere with lactation involved over five hundred women and their feeding patterns with their first baby. Among those mothers who breastfed for at least two months, the average nursing period was considerably shorter for smokers than for nonsmokers. Among these five hundred women were some who had given up smoking during pregnancy. The length of time they continued to nurse was similar to that of women who had never smoked. In this study the mothers were not asked their reasons for stopping breastfeeding so although suggestive, it cannot be assumed that an inadequate milk supply was the cause.

Overall, the information relating smoking and nursing is very sparse and to a considerable degree inconclusive. The limited data that are available do suggest that smoking may interfere with lactation and that some of the nicotine is transmitted to the baby via the milk. Whether or not this nicotine has a harmful effect upon the infant is a question that remains to be answered.

chapter ten
Long-term Effects

Normal development of the fetus depends upon a complicated interaction of both genetic and nongenetic factors. Probably the most critical period in the developmental process occurs during organogenesis—the first eight weeks after the formation of the zygote, when the organs of the body begin to develop. During this period the orderly sequence of development can be disrupted severely by errors in the genetic makeup of the embryo, by conditions of the environment to which it is exposed, or by both kinds of element acting together.

That abnormalities of the fetus can be produced by substances ingested by the mother during pregnancy has been known for a long time. The experience with Thalidomide served to focus attention on this matter. The list of harmful products is large. Synthetic progesterone (a sex hormone) has caused masculinization of female infants. Diethylstilbesterol (DES, another synthetic sex hormone) taken during pregnancy is associated with a rare form of vaginal cancer in young women whose mothers received the drug. Diazepam (Valium), a tranquilizer, administered during labor results in infants who are apathetic, have a low temperature, feed poorly, and suffer spells of shallow breathing. The use of excessive amounts of aspirin has led to bleeding disorders in infants. Drugs containing iodine can cause congenital goiter in the baby. The drinking of alcohol, at both an alcoholic and a heavy social level, may alter the behavior of the infant.

Smoking of cigarettes during pregnancy has its own influence on the newborn, as we have seen, and may even affect the older baby. Such effects will be described in this chapter.

One thing is clear: the placenta is not an absolute barrier and does not protect the fetus. Therefore, when drugs are to be administered to the pregnant woman, the safety of the fetus must be a prime consideration. The effects of a harmful agent may be of major significance, easily and quickly detected at birth. Or they may be subtle, becoming evident only years later. An example of this phenomenon is an impairment in the ability to learn, which sometimes becomes apparent only when the child enters school.

A teratogen is a substance capable of producing abnormalities during intrauterine development that may show themselves before birth, at birth, or later in life. Clinical evidence and experimental work on animals have revealed several principles regarding these agents.

It is known that embryos are not equally responsive to the action of a teratogen. In their susceptibility to harmful prenatal influences great differences exist both between embryos of the same species and between embryos of different species. The fact that a drug can cause an abnormality in an animal does not mean that it can do the same in humans.

The effect that a teratogen has on an embryo depends to a large extent on when in pregnancy it acts. For a week or so after fertilization, before the embryo is embedded in the wall of the uterus and before the process of organ formation has begun, a harmful agent often has an all or nothing effect. Either the embryo is unharmed or it dies. Rarely do teratogens applied during this period cause gross structural abnormalities.

The most critical period for the embryo is the interval between implantation and the end of the first three months of pregnancy. This is the time when the most active and rapid cellular proliferation takes place, when the rudiments of the organ systems are laid down, and when the primary tissues begin to differentiate from each other and development takes place. A harmful agent, by slowing down or stopping completely the process of differentiation, even for a short time, or by disrupting the orderly sequence of development can produce marked deviations from the normal and lead to malformations of various organs.

Formerly it was believed that the type of malformation produced by a prenatal disturbance depended solely on when in pregnancy the insult occurred; in other words, those parts of the body undergoing critical development at the moment were damaged, regardless of the noxious agent. According to this principle, all teratogens, if applied at exactly the same stage of pregnancy, would produce the identical malformation. This idea is no longer accepted. Both the specific harmful agent and the time during pregnancy that it is applied play a significant part in determining which kinds of abnormality are produced. Applied at the same stage of pregnancy, different teratogens can cause diverse malformations.

The remainder of the pregnancy is a period mainly of growth of parts of the body whose structure and function have already been established. No new organs are laid down. During this time few congenital malformations are produced by teratogens. Rather, teratogens can cause abnormal growth of various structures.

The human brain differs from other tissues and organs in that its development is not complete at the end of pregnancy but goes on after birth. Because of the supreme importance of the brain, in periods of deprivation the body has a brain-sparing mechanism. Blood, carrying oxygen and food, will be shunted away from less vital organs and rerouted to the brain. For example, in severe cases of malnutrition during pregnancy, the body of the newborn infant may be smaller than normal, whereas the brain may approximate the size of that of a well-fed child. As a result, a malnourished newborn frequently appears to have a disproportionately large head. But even with this protective mechanism the brain and the rest of the nervous system can be targets of damaging substances.

The newborn infant can withstand a certain interval of lowered levels of oxygen and survive. However, long-term follow-ups have shown that a considerable number of these infants in whom the period of hypoxia (oxygen deficiency) has been relatively short show disorders of the nervous system at a later age. Some of these babies develop cerebral palsy or childhood epilepsy or exhibit mental retardation or the syndrome of minimal brain dysfunction. This last group includes infants, children, and adolescents who have behavioral disorders often accompanied by learning defects, difficulty in reading, hyperactivity, motor disturbances such as awkwardness, abnormal neurologic patterns, and electro-encephalographic irregularities. The baby of low birth weight is especially susceptible to hypoxic brain damage.

There appears to be no doubt that smoking in pregnancy has certain short-term risks for the fetus, such as retardation of intrauterine growth. However, the question as to whether smoking has any permanent effects on the child has not been answered clearly. The modern and increasing concern for the prevention of long-term neurologic and intellectual handicaps in children has prompted attempts to identify factors that may adversely affect fetal growth and development. One of these factors may be smoking.

In previous chapters the evidence has been described relating cigarette smoking to effects on the fetus that can be seen at birth or within a few days afterward. It is of equal if not greater importance to know whether the observations and measurements taken at birth disappear as the child gets older or whether maternal smoking during pregnancy has long-term consequences for the child as he or she grows. The mechanisms that may retard fetal growth may also influence later mental functioning or various other behaviors. Several investigators have attempted to determine whether there are such long-term effects upon the physical growth, intellectual development, and emotional status of the children of maternal smokers.

Studying the long-term effects of maternal smoking is not as easy as it might first appear. There is the practical problem of keeping in touch with the children for several years so that repeated measurements can be taken of whatever effect may be of interest to the investigator. There is also the serious problem that many events unrelated to maternal smoking occur during the growth of the child that may well influence the very things the researcher is interested in linking to smoking. This makes the interpretation of any results a complex matter. For these reasons the long-term effects of smoking during pregnancy are less well documented than some of the findings described in earlier chapters.

One of the earliest studies, published in 1968, reported the results of examining fifteen hundred infants several times between birth and one year of age. The researchers were interested in testing the following hypothesis: if smoking by the mother is acting as a low-grade poison and thereby retarding fetal growth, the smaller babies born to these smokers might be expected to grow more quickly after birth once away from the influence of the smoke. Measurements of the weight gained and increases in head circumference in the babies of smokers and nonsmokers were compared at six weeks, six months, and one year after birth. It was found that the rate of weight gain and the increase in head circumference were indeed greater among the smokers' babies up to the sixth month. However, this spurt ceased by the first year, and at this age the infants born to maternal smokers tended to be lighter than those born to nonsmoking mothers.

The first investigations of whether factors underlying the lessened fetal growth may also have long-term risks were first reported in the early 1970s. The suspicion was that if diminished availability of oxygen is a significant contributing factor in the lowered birth weight, then this same hypoxia could be causing other alterations, including mild brain damage, that may show up only when the infant is somewhat older.

In 1972 data from approximately five thousand pregnancies were collected from women living in Baltimore's inner city. Women who had smoked at least ten cigarettes every day from the beginning of pregnancy were compared with nonsmokers. Of the women, eighty-eight smokers and eighty-eight nonsmokers were matched so as to be similar with respect to age, race, educational background, time of delivery, and sex of the baby. Their children were examined several times until the age of seven. At birth, the babies of the smokers were on the average approximately nine ounces lighter and just under an inch shorter than the infants of nonsmokers. These birth results are in agreement with those from the many studies we described earlier. The differences in weight and body length were still evident when the two groups of babies were compared at one year of age. However, when the children were examined at four years the differences were no longer observed. Nor were any differences found when the children were given a variety of standard intelligence tests. The similarity among the children of smokers and nonsmokers on physical measurements and intellectual functioning was also evident when the youngsters were measured for a third time at seven years of age, although a slight trend favoring the nonsmokers' children was observed on the intelligence tests.

Several researchers have suggested that the study just described be interpreted with caution because only eighty-eight pairs of children were examined. It has been argued that the physical and intellectual long-term effects of maternal smoking may be so subtle that differences would be noted only if a large number of boys and girls were examined. More recent work tends to back this point of view, although considerably more research and information are needed before this issue can be settled.

In 1973, two scientists examined data from seventeen

thousand children. These were virtually all the babies born in England, Scotland, and Wales in a one-week period during 1958. Reading was tested at the age of seven and reading, mathematics, and general ability were examined when the children were eleven. Physical measurements were also made at these two ages. Consistent differences in height and reading ability were found between the children of smokers and nonsmokers at ages seven and eleven, and the differences increased with the number of cigarettes smoked during pregnancy. On average the children of mothers who had smoked ten or more cigarettes each day were approximately half an inch shorter and between three and five months slower in reading, mathematics, and general ability as compared to the children of nonsmokers. These findings were still observed consistently when allowances for social and biological differences between the smoking and nonsmoking groups were made. These effects of maternal smoking are small compared to other influences such as social class and the number of other children in the family; nevertheless, the findings do suggest a continuing effect of smoking during pregnancy.

In 1976 a Canadian report was published that described children of two types of low birth weight and compared them to normal birth weight infants. The low birth weight babies were eighty-one small for dates infants and ninety-nine babies who were defined as premature by having a gestation period of less than thirty-seven weeks. These babies were compared to 146 normal birth weight infants, with the smoking histories of all mothers being taken. As one might expect from the investigations described in Chapter 7 there were disproportionately more smokers among the mothers of the small for dates infants. The babies were followed up for several years. At the age of six and a half, the children of nonsmoking mothers in all three categories averaged approximately one half to three fourths of an inch taller and one to three pounds heavier than children of smoking mothers.

The most consistent differences were noted among the normal birth weight children of smoking and nonsmoking mothers. In a series of psychological tests, the average scores in the three categories were nearly always higher among the nonsmokers' children. The findings from both the physical growth patterns and the intelligence measures are similar to those in the large British study described previously.

Growth and cognitive development have not been the only long-term effects of smoking examined. The possible consequences of maternal smoking on the behavior of the child have also been considered. Recently an association between smoking during pregnancy and hyperactivity, one of the most widespread of children's disorders, has been proposed. Simply defined, hyperactivity is a long-term childhood pattern characterized by excessive restlessness and inattentiveness with associated problems of conduct and learning disabilities. For a proper diagnosis it is critically important that the behavioral history of the child be known. Hyperactivity shows itself as a persistent pattern of excessive activity in situations that require suppression of certain movements. The term "persistent" must be emphasized. Typically, this disorder shows itself first between the ages of two and six and begins to fade during adolescence. During childhood, the pattern of the absence of movement inhibition is consistent year after year.

Very often it is in a classroom setting that a hyperactive child is recognized. The reason for this is that such behavior is most evident in situations in which the boy or girl is required to be attentive and relatively still.

A group of Canadian workers compared the maternal smoking habits of mothers of twenty hyperactive children, mothers of twenty children who were not hyperactive but who were being treated at a clinic for reading difficulties, and mothers of twenty children with no apparent disorders. Each hyperactive child was matched with a child in the other two groups by age, sex, and social class. Differences in the smoking habits of the mothers were striking and suggestive. Mothers of the hyperactive children had consumed more than twice as many cigarettes during pregnancy as had the women in the other two groups. In fact, sixteen out of the twenty women who had hyperactive children smoked during pregnancy. Although not mentioned in the report of this study it can be presumed, from national averages, that smokers in the other two groups numbered approximately six to eight out of twenty.

The researchers interpreted their findings in the following fashion. They, and others, feel that one of the underlying causes of hyperactivity is slight damage to certain parts of the brain. Such damage could result from a reduced supply of oxygen during pregnancy, which, as indicated earlier, is an effect associated with smoking.

Obviously these data are of a most preliminary nature and at best are only suggestive. However, they certainly deserve consideration and this thesis warrants further investigation.

The studies described in this chapter represent the present state of knowledge with respect to the long-term effects of smoking. It is obvious that the information is relatively limited and firm conclusions cannot be made at this time. However, the available evidence does lean toward the contention that there are long-term unfavorable effects associated with maternal smoking. Unfortunately for the woman who is presently pregnant or who is considering having children we cannot be more definitive.

chapter eleven
Conclusions and Alternatives

During pregnancy mother, placenta, and fetus—one old and two new, distinct biological systems—combine in a marvelously intricate fashion to produce, at the end of nine months, a new being ready for the outside world. Although these three systems do exhibit a tremendous amount of interdependency each has a particular role to play during pregnancy and each reacts in a somewhat different manner and to a somewhat different degree to potentially harmful substances or events.

For a long time it has been accepted that the pregnant woman and her unborn baby are particularly susceptible to the effects of outside influences. Outside influences, or environmental factors as they are often called, include drugs, diseases, and stress. Until fairly recently the developing baby was considered to be at the same risk level as the mother, but unfortunate experience has resulted in the changing of that opinion. We now know that the fetus must be considered separately from the mother as far as vulnerability is concerned.

Diseases as mild as German measles, if contracted in the early months of pregnancy, while having no direct effect upon the mother-to-be, may cause defects such as malformation of the heart, cataracts of the eyes, and deafness in the newborn. Experience with the drug Thalidomide tragically demonstrated fetal vulnerability. This drug, a mild sedative, was in part originally advocated because it was so safe for most of the population. Doses of up to ten or fifteen times the recommended level could be taken by adults and even children without marked side effects. Unfortunately, the same was not true for the unborn baby. In some instances even a single normal dose taken by a pregnant woman caused severe malformations in the fetus. If Thalidomide was taken during the fifth to the seventh week of pregnancy it could cause effects that are all too well known today: absence of the long bones of the arms and legs, causing the deformed hands and feet to be close to the trunk, giving a flipperlike look to the limbs. These tragic examples provide a painful lesson. They illustrate in a rather extreme manner that the fetus can be harmed by environmental factors whose effects cannot be predicted on the basis of the mother's response to such factors.

The most likely reason for this vulnerability in the unborn baby is that the period from conception until birth is the time of most rapid growth and of tissue and organ specialization. During this nine-month period the baby increases in weight two billion times while changing from a single cell into a complex being. It is not surprising that as these enormous changes occur, environmental influences may produce potent and possibly long-lasting effects.

A perusal of recent professional articles on the topic of child development or a trip to the appropriate section in a library reveals that a widely followed current approach in the study of the development of children is to examine the role of very early experiences. This approach has come about because of the realization that if we can establish how and what factors affect young children we are in a better position to shape the environment to which our children are exposed.

The evidence discussed in this book leads clearly to the conclusion that the by-products of smoking are one set of environmental factors that have adverse consequences for the unborn child. It follows that the appropriate time to begin to control this particular environmental factor is the critical prenatal period.

In recent surveys 90 percent of adults stated that smoking is harmful to their own bodies. However, less than two-thirds of young women who smoked felt that smoking during pregnancy can be harmful to the unborn child. This gap in knowledge reflects the relative neglect of pregnant women as a target group for antismoking efforts. Why is this so? Certainly part of the answer lies in the fact that until recently the effects of smoking on the unborn were not as clearly established or described in the scientific literature as were the effects of smoking on the lungs. We hope that the evidence presented in the previous chapters points clearly to the conclusion that the smoking of cigarettes by a pregnant woman has a considerable detrimental effect upon the fetus.

The major points that we have explored in the book can be highlighted as follows:

Smoking cigarettes while pregnant can adversely affect many stages of the life of the child—the fetus, the newborn, the infant, and beyond. During the pregnancy the potential problems associated with smoking range from an increased risk of complications that can result in the loss of the baby to a slowing in fetal growth as seen in reduced body weight, shortened body length, and smaller head circumference. At birth and during the first few days of life the evidence suggests that smoking during pregnancy increases the likelihood of mild disorders of the nervous system as reflected in tremors, irritability, and a decreased tendency to ignore repetitive stimulation. Subtle hearing impairments and interference with nursing also are consequences associated with smoking during pregnancy that appear during infancy. Finally, there is some evidence that smoking may have long-term effects on the child. Reduced physical growth, slightly poorer performance on intelligence tests, and some behavioral disorders in the child of school age have all been linked to cigarette use during pregnancy.

As we have seen, some of these complications and

adverse outcomes are not definitely linked to smoking, but there is enough convincing evidence to state most emphatically that cigarette use during pregnancy can no longer be regarded as medically inconsequential. The possibility that smoking harms the unborn child is great enough that, from a preventive point of view, a very strong case can be made for stopping the habit.

Although it is best for a woman never to have smoked or to have given up cigarettes for a considerable length of time prior to her pregnancy, two points raised in several chapters must be reemphasized. First, for almost every risk factor associated with maternal smoking there appears to be a dose response relationship. That is, the more cigarettes a woman smokes the greater the probability that the baby will be affected. This means that even if smoking cannot be given up entirely a reduction in the number of cigarettes smoked would reduce the likelihood of the habit's adversely affecting the unborn child. Decreasing the amount of cigarettes smoked also reduces the severity of the effects that may be caused by smoking. The second point that we wish to raise again is somewhat more controversial. This involves the timing of giving up or reducing the cigarette habit. A number of large studies have found that giving up smoking even as late as the beginning of the second trimester of pregnancy reduces the likelihood of many of the adverse effects upon the developing baby. However, a recent American study disputes this claim; the data suggested that smoking even in the year before pregnancy increases the risk to the fetus. Although this issue remains to be resolved researchers working in the area of pregnancy and smoking agree that the best way to reduce the risk of cigarettes' affecting the unborn baby is for the mother to give up smoking as much before the birth as possible. If a pregnancy is planned the best way for a smoker to minimize the risk to the fetus is to give up cigarettes well before becoming pregnant.

Even if the smoking woman is convinced that the

cigarette habit has serious undesirable effects for the unborn baby the solution to the problem is far from simple. Giving up cigarettes or even reducing the number smoked is for most people no small task. In earlier sections of the book when we talked about the constituents of cigarette smoke (Chapter 3) and about the newborn baby (Chapter 8), the physiological dependence that develops on nicotine and the symptoms that accompany its withdrawal were discussed. This is one important factor that the smoker must overcome but it is not the major one. The withdrawal symptoms usually disappear within a week if no cigarettes are used yet many smokers weeks or months later—well after the physiological craving for nicotine has passed—return to their old habits. In other words, psychological and not physiological factors frequently play the critical role in determining the success or failure of giving up cigarettes. This is a very important point in the consideration of smoking and pregnancy and we will return to it several times in this chapter.

As we mentioned earlier, virtually all adults are aware that smoking is not good for one's health, yet still more than one in three lights up regularly. So, for many women, knowing smoking is harmful is not sufficient motivation to stop. Now, if we add the argument to mothers-to-be or women thinking of having a child that smoking is a hazard to the baby's health we add a strong incentive for at no other time during a woman's life is there likely to be a greater sense of responsibility for another human life than during pregnancy. Of course, it is easier to give this advice than to take it, but there is the important psychological point that the more positive reasons a person can see for changing behavior, even if they value the particular behavior, the more likely they are to change. The strength of the desire to change is perhaps the key factor in determining the success or failure of attempts to stop smoking. We will get back to this point later, but now the point we wish to make is that this makes

113

mothers-to-be good candidates for such a behavioral change provided they are well informed.

Over thirty million North Americans stopped smoking between 1965 and 1980. About 90 percent of these people did so without any organized smoking cessation program. The others gave up smoking by taking part in special clinics that use hypnosis, behavior modification, medication, or group therapy. No matter what approach is taken, some specific procedures or self-imposed rules must be followed by the smoker in order to be successful. It is not the purpose of this book to provide a detailed discussion of various ways that have been used to kick the habit. However, we will suggest some general steps that may be useful for smokers who are or plan to become pregnant.

It must be kept in mind that there are tremendous variations among individuals and what may work for one may not for another. The same applies to bodily and mental reactions that may occur following the giving up of a long-standing cigarette habit. Obviously, an important component that affects both the degree of difficulty in giving up cigarettes and the cravings and other side effects that may follow is how long one has smoked and what the daily cigarette intake has been. As with any well-established pattern of behavior, the longer the habit has existed and the stronger it has been, the harder it will be to give it up.

The first step in modifying any behavior, including the cigarette habit, is to get an accurate picture of the behavior one intends to change. In the case of smoking what must be estalished is how many cigarettes are consumed daily, in what situations, and with what consequences. There are many ways that this can be done. Perhaps the easiest and most direct procedure is a frequency check made by the mother-to-be on a small piece of paper carried in her cigarette package. Not only should the number of cigarettes smoked be recorded but also, in two or three words, the reason for lighting up or the situation in which smoking occurred. This information, gathered over a period of time, may reveal patterns that the smoker may not have noticed. For example, if smoking occurs in particular situations such as during television commercials or after meals, then alternate activities that are incompatible with smoking can be planned for these periods.

Broadly speaking, the reasons for smoking can be divided into two general categories: smoking in response to some inner need and smoking for social reasons. Several specific factors have been identified that appear to influence smokers to continue: (1) stimulation—getting a sense of increased energy; (2) manipulation—getting satisfaction from lighting and handling cigarettes; (3) pleasurable relaxation—rewarding oneself with a cigarette after the need to stay alert and tense has passed or facilitating social interaction; (4) habit—not missing cigarettes if they are not available but automatically lighting up if they are to hand or if they are offered (the smoker does not think that the cigarettes make her feel different); (5) reduction of negative feelings—smoking in order to cope with undesirable emotions such as tension, anxiety, or anger in difficult situations; and (6) addiction—smoking to prevent the strong, unpleasant sense of craving that being without cigarettes produces or the associated concern of overeating if smoking is stopped. Some smokers may feel that one of these factors is the main reason for their habit but most individuals have many reasons for smoking.

The little slip of paper we suggested that smokers keep in their cigarette packages will very often identify the factor or factors that lead to the continuation of the habit and the situations in which cigarettes are smoked. If this is the case the next step is to consider alternatives that could counteract the need to smoke.

Among women in general, and presumably also among mothers-to-be, it has been found that the impetus to continue smoking frequently revolves around two of the reasons mentioned above: the need to cope with feelings of tension produced by stress or anger, for example, and the concern that weight gain will follow the stopping of smoking.

Let's deal with the eating issue first. A belief held by about 60 percent of both smokers and nonsmokers is that once a longtime cigarette habit is stopped the appetite will increase and pounds will be put on. In fact, this does appear to be the case for a few weeks after stopping, but typically within a month the situation changes. National health statistics indicate that one-third of all smokers who quit lose weight, one-third have no weight change at all, and one-third gain weight. It is the consensus of experts that this latter group may be using food as an oral pacifier and is eating food quite indiscriminately.

If weight gain is of concern to a mother-to-be who is a smoker a number of points must be considered. First of all, it has been estimated that smoking a package of cigarettes a day puts as much strain on one's body as weighing an extra sixty pounds. This figure makes the slight weight gain that often occurs immediately after quitting relatively insignificant. A second point with respect to weight gain is the idea of planning aspects of one's diet after one stops smoking. This planning should be completed before giving up cigarettes; thinking in advance is an important component of a successful campaign to stop smoking.

A number of foods should be avoided, including the junk foods commonly eaten when cigarettes are smoked, such as potato chips, pretzels, soft drinks, french fries, candies, and cookies. These foods have little or no nutritional value but are laden with calories. In the bowls or dishes that normally contain such snack foods the mother-to-be might place raw fruit and vegetables: chopped up carrots, cauliflower pieces, mushrooms, celery, nuts, raisins, and sunflower seeds make excellent and tasty nibbly foods. Snacks in this form serve a number of useful purposes, some of which are not obvious at first glance. Certainly they are nutritious. But beyond that they help rid the body of waste materials, which in turn helps keep the weight down. Reaching for and nibbling such food also has the added benefit of keeping the former smoker busy with her fingers when they might otherwise be occupied with lighting up a cigarette. Finally, by changing her snack foods, the woman weakens a link between her living style and smoking. For if she nibbled on food that in the past was eaten while she smoked, the snack would serve as a constant reminder of cigarettes. By eliminating the snacks one associates with smoking, the habit is less likely to return.

Another group of foods that one ought to cut down on once smoking has been stopped are coffee, tea, and colas. All of these contain caffeine, a substance that strongly stimulates the nervous system. Such stimulation may well bring on a heightened desire for a cigarette to "settle the nerves" and the habit becomes that much harder to break. Fruit juices have been found by many to be a good substitute for caffeine containing drinks.

Very often cigarettes and alcohol are consumed at the same time. The calorie content of most alcoholic drinks is quite high and potentially this can be a problem. First of all, pregnant women must not substitute alcohol for cigarettes. Regular drinking during pregnancy is definitely risky. A couple of drinks a day or an occasional binge has been associated with adverse effects upon the unborn baby. However, if the mother-to-be does not wish to give up alcohol completely, sticking to light beers, with their fewer calories, is one way to get around the fattening aspect of alcohol. Another possibility is to replace liquors such as gin or rye with table wines, as a glass of the latter contains approximately 85 calories whereas a shot of most liquors contains 105 calories.

During the first few days after stopping smoking one of the symptoms reported by some women is an uneasy feeling in the stomach. This sensation is judged by some to be a sign of hunger. It is not. Rather, it is one of the adjustments the digestive system has to make in the absence of the constituents of smoke. Drinking some water or fruit juice when this sensation arises is frequently helpful.

Coupled with watching one's food habits, an increase in activity or exercise will almost certainly prevent weight gain. Not only does activity burn up calories but it also speeds up the adjustment of the body to its new nicotine-free state. It is quite easy for a woman to increase her activity, say, through regular exercise such as swimming or bicycle riding or through consciously doing more of everyday things such as walking briskly around the house, walking up or down a flight or two of stairs instead of taking the elevator, lifting up the arms and stretching, or parking the car or getting off the bus a block before her destination.

Even moderate activity or exercise has a marked role in deciding whether calories are or are not going to be reflected as a gain in weight. For example, if one lies down after eating a slice of apple pie or drinking a milk shake, the body will take about five hours to burn off the four hundred calories contained in either item. Those calories could be worked off by two hours of bowling, an hour and a half of ironing, just over an hour of walking, fifty minutes of bicycle riding, or half an hour of swimming. The 115 calories contained in a slice of bread could be utilized by lying down for ninety minutes, by thirty-five minutes of bowling, less than half an hour of ironing, twenty minutes of walking, fourteen minutes of bicycling, or ten minutes of swimming. A woman who puts together a small increase in physical activity with a small reduction in caloric intake can significantly reduce her weight.

Not only does activity in any form help get rid of calories but also it is a useful and effective way of controlling one of the other major reasons why women continue to smoke, that is, to cope with tension. Stress and strong emotions produce an increase in adrenalin. This hormone, produced by the adrenal glands, lying near the kidneys, travels throughout the body. Its function is to get the organs and the nervous system in a state of readiness to respond to whatever caused the strong emotions. One of the consequences of the release of adrenalin is a general feeling of tension. Activity, in the form of even mild physical exertion, uses up some of the adrenalin and helps to reduce tension. In this way exercise can be effective when the need for a tension relieving cigarette is felt. Another alternative to the tension reducing properties associated by some women with cigarette smoking is a leisurely bath. Warm water soothes, loosens muscles, and increases blood flow, physiological changes that help calm one.

Some women report that the desire for a cigarette is strong just before going to sleep for the night. Many smokers feel this ritual helps them unwind before sleeping. An alternative to smoking at this time is the drinking of a warm glass of milk. This age-old sleep remedy has a soothing effect on jangled nerves and thus is particularly useful during the first few days after cigarettes have been given up.

There is considerable controversy as to whether it is better gradually to reduce the amount smoked or to give up cigarettes all at once—so-called cold turkey. Arguments can be made for both approaches. Stopping the habit completely and suddenly has many psychological advantages. For example, things that might tempt the smoker to light up or that remind the woman of cigarettes can be gotten rid of. She can make sure that there are no cigarettes in her purse or around the home, thus making it somewhat harder to have "just one." Ashtrays, books of matches, and other material closely linked to smoking can also be removed. Out of sight, out of mind has some truth to it. On the other hand, if the gradual reduction approach is taken the body can adjust to the lowered nicotine levels somewhat more easily than if nicotine is eliminated all at once. So, physiologically the reduction procedure has its advantages but psychologically going cold turkey might be easier.

A combination of both approaches might be the answer

for many women. This would involve setting a date in the fairly immediate future—say, three weeks down the road—when smoking will be stopped entirely. Between the setting of the date and the critical day itself the smoker can gradually cut down on the number of cigarettes smoked perhaps by not smoking in one or two particular situations that she normally smoked in. This breaking in period has a number of advantages. One can pick the critical day to be a day when no other stressful events such as a move, a deadline at work, or giving a party are expected. The woman can also use this period to develop alternate activities and to adopt eating habits that will be followed once smoking is given up entirely.

In Chapter 8 we discussed the psychological and physiological disturbances that frequently occur following the cessation of smoking. The symptoms and their strength will differ from individual to individual. Restlessness, sleep disturbance, and drowsiness may be felt for the first few days. As mentioned before, warm milk at bedtime often helps the new nonsmoker to fall asleep. It is not uncommon to feel unusually sleepy during the day for a while after giving up cigarettes. Planning for occasional naps or extra sleep during the first week or so is a sensible way of dealing with this particular withdrawal symptom.

Occasional dizziness, slight tremors, and headaches may be experienced by women giving up smoking. These symptoms are thought to be associated in part with the body's getting used to reduced levels of carbon monoxide. In other words, even though carbon monoxide is a highly undesirable by-product of smoke inhalation, the body has adapted itself to this substance and exhibits withdrawal symptoms in its absence. A suggested way to relieve these symptoms is deep breathing and mild exercise so as to increase the inhalation of oxygen. It would also be beneficial, for the same reason, to keep the bedroom windows open at night.

Although a heavy smoker who stops her habit will

most likely experience some of the symptoms we have just described, surprisingly the key factor in determining the success or failure of quitting cigarettes is probably not the extent or severity of withdrawal symptoms. More important is the intensity of the desire that underlies the decision to stop smoking. The important role of motivation becomes evident when the results of various formal programs to stop smoking are examined. All approaches show very similar short- and long-term results. For example, many programs report that about 70 percent of those who begin treatment actually stop smoking initially. A significant number of those who do stop unfortunately resume smoking within the first six months and by twelve months over half of those who gave up cigarettes have gone back to their old habit. After the first year the rate of people who return to smoking slows down considerably. Several researchers have observed that the succes rate is somewhat lower among women than men. However, the women in question were not pregnant. What the rate of failure is among mothers-to-be is an unanswered question at this time.

The similarity among the wide array of approaches indicates that the success or failure rate is independent of the strategy used to break the habit. What appears to happen is that the desire to stop smoking, which presumably is similar among smokers in every treatment, swamps the effects of whatever technique is being used. Thus, smokers with the highest motivation in each of the treatment approaches are successful whereas smokers at the other end of the motivational scale are not.

These statistics indicating the vital role of motivation in successfully giving up cigarettes serve as a very strong argument for giving pregnant smokers and women who are thinking of having children as much information as is known about smoking and pregnancy. This information may well provide the woman with the powerful incentive needed to stop smoking if she so chooses.

Prenatal classes are a well-accepted part of public health programs and are found in most communities in North America. These classes are widely attended. In 1978–1979 in the Ottawa area over 75 percent of mothers interviewed had attended a prenatal class during one of their pregnancies. Instructors in these classes calm the fears of couples by providing an accurate description of pregnancy and childbirth and refuting popular misconceptions. They teach couples how to deal with labor and delivery, accentuate the positive, and emphasize that childbearing is essentially a normal process. This philosophy, which is also evident among physicians, has perhaps caused a downplaying of the negative features of being pregnant. The powerful advertising techniques that equate the act of smoking with women's liberation, maturity, and sexual allure (all in the same breath) have enticed young women into the smokers' ranks at a faster rate than any other group. Prenatal classes might be one forum in which the message of the advertisers can be counteracted. Naturally, discussion of this subject may be disconcerting to the mother-to-be who smokes but this initial feeling is bound to lessen when the woman understands the benefits to her future child that stopping or reducing smoking as early in pregnancy as possible can produce. The woman who is exposed to such information during her first pregnancy may decide to stop smoking well in advance of future pregnancies and thereby minimize the risk to future babies.

As we noted in various chapters, the components of tobacco smoke cross from mother to unborn child via the placenta and enter the circulatory system of the fetus. There are short-term effects on the fetus, on the newborn, and on the young baby and possible long-term effects that carry over into childhood. Furthermore, if the baby is already at risk because of some other known or unknown factors, smoking may be the straw that breaks the camel's back. Faced with this state of affairs the woman who smokes and who is considering having a baby or who is already pregnant must make a critical decision. Giving up smoking requires, in almost all cases, considerable self-sacrifice. The smoking woman is most likely well aware of this fact and the anxieties and stress that stopping the cigarette habit may bring. We hope our book provides that woman with sufficient information about the other side of the issue. She is the one who must make the decision and carry it through.

Glossary

Abruptio Placenta

A premature separation of the placenta from the wall of the uterus.

Addiction

Compulsive use of habit-forming drugs.

Adrenal Glands

A complex pair of endocrine glands placed just above the kidneys. They make hormones that affect all bodily functions but are concerned principally in helping to keep the internal environment of the body constant.

Adrenalin or Epinephrine

A hormone secreted by the adrenal glands. It is a potent stimulator of the sympathetic nervous system, which can increase blood pressure and heart rate.

Amniotic Fluid

A fluid derived primarily from a filtrate of the mother's blood and in which the embryo floats. The volume at term is between one and two pints.

Anemia

A condition in which the blood is deficient in red blood cells, in hemoglobin, or in total volume. Frequently the symptoms include a lack of vitality.

Anoxia

A state in which the body is deprived of oxygen.

Antibody

A product of the body's reaction to an outside influence.

Should a foreign protein get into the body, the cells make antibodies that will destroy the protein.

Apgar

A numerical assessment of the condition of a newborn infant made at one minute and again at five minutes after birth; this rating is the sum of points assigned to the following five items: (1) heart rate; (2) respiratory effort; (3) muscle tone; (4) reflex irritability; and (5) color.

Ascorbic Acid

See Vitamin C.

Asphyxia

A condition caused by lack of oxygen in the lungs and in the body's cells, which may result in death.

Calorie

A unit of energy. The number of daily calories required to carry on the processes necessary for life in an adult is approximately sixteen hundred; for hard, continuous work, about four thousand calories daily. During pregnancy approximately two hundred calories per day above the usual adequate diet are needed.

Carbon Monoxide

One of the gaseous products of smoking that, by combining with the hemoglobin in the blood, can limit the amount of oxygen carried to tissues.

Carboxyhemoglobin

The result of carbon monoxide's combining with hemoglobin. The formation of carboxyhemoglobin results in a displacement of oxygen from hemoglobin.

Cardiovascular

Involving the heart and blood vessels.

Cervix

The narrow outer end of the uterus located partly above and partly within the vagina.

Cleft Palate

A congenital narrow split of the roof of the mouth that very often is combined with harelip.

Clinical Significance

A situation where the measurement taken alters behavior or physiology to the extent that it affects the individual's life style.

Cold Turkey

An abrupt cessation of drug intake that is usually accompanied by symptoms of withdrawal.

Colostrum

The thin, yellow, milky fluid secreted by the mammary glands a few days before and after birth.

Congenital

Referring to deformities, diseases, etc., that are either present at birth or, being transmitted directly from the parents, show themselves after birth.

Diffusion

The process of spreading out. Diffusion is a passive process not requiring metabolic energy from cells. It is important in the movement of some materials across the placenta.

Drug Dependency

State in which the use of a drug is necessary for either physical or psychological well-being.

Electroencephalography

Measurement of the electrical activity of the brain. The electroencephalogram, or EEG, usually measured over several minutes or longer, is useful for research purposes and clinical diagnosis.

Embryo

A developing baby—for humans during the first eight weeks of intrauterine existence, during which period the organs are being formed.

Endocrine Gland

A gland that discharges chemical substances known as hormones directly into the blood stream which then carries them to all parts of the body, resulting in many kinds of physiological changes.

Enzyme

Chemicals existing in cells that speed up reactions such as the utilization of oxygen and the breaking down of foodstuffs. Enzymes remain unchanged during their participation in chemical reactions.

Epinephrine

See Adrenalin.

Estrogen

A female sex hormone formed primarily in the ovaries. It is responsible for the development of the female sex characteristics and plays an important role in producing an environment suitable for the fertilization, implantation, and nutrition of the early embryo.

Fallopian Tubes

These tubes, one on each side of the pelvic cavity, are attached at one end to the uterus and have the other unattached but lying close to the ovary. The tubes conduct the egg from the ovaries to the interior of the uterus.

Fertilized Ovum

The egg from the female after its union with male sperm.

Fetus

A developing baby—for humans during the last thirty-two weeks of intrauterine life, during which period the organ structures laid down in the earlier (embryonic) stage are developed.

Gene

A tiny substance, grouped into chromosomes, that directs the growth of cells into specific parts of the body and accounts for inherited individual differences.

Harelip

A congenital cleft or division in the upper lip.

Hemoglobin

An iron-containing protein in the red blood cells that is capable of carrying oxygen to the tissues.

Hormones

These substances act as chemical messengers in the blood, stimulating the body's cells to perform their functions. They influence growth, metabolism, and milk production and secretion, for example.

Hyperactivity

A long-term childhood pattern characterized by persistent, excessive restlessness and inattentiveness and associated problems of conduct and learning difficulty.

Hypothalamus

An important structure in the brain that has a large influence on the pituitary gland.

Involuntary Smoking

The inhalation by a nonsmoker of the products contained in the atomsphere of a smoke-filled environment.

Lobules of the Breast

These structures are major subdivisions of the secreting portion of the mammary gland; each is drained by a single lactiferous duct.

Mainstream Smoke

Smoke that is exhaled by smokers after they have drawn it through the cigarette.

Meconium

The brown, semi-fluid material that collects in the bowels of a baby before birth and ought to be discharged at the time of birth or shortly afterwards.

Moro Reflex

This reflex is set off in the newborn by a sudden motion. The reflex starts off with a startle: the baby throws out his or her arms and often cries out; having extended the arms the baby then brings them together with the effect of clasping anyone who might be within reach.

Motor Behavior

Behavior resulting from the activity of muscles and nerves that produces a movement.

Organogenesis

The development or growth of organs.

Ova

Female reproductive cells (the singular is ovum), which after fertilization develop into new members of the same species.

Ovary
One of the two sexual glands in which the ova are formed.

Oxytocin
A hormone secreted by the posterior portion of the pituitary gland. This substance allows the milk ducts in the breasts to release milk through the nipples and also causes contraction of the uterus.

Oxytocinase
An enzyme produced by the placenta that inhibits the action of oxytocin and thereby inhibits premature labor.

Passive Smoking
See Involuntary Smoking.

Perinatal
The period of time that includes late pregnancy and the first week after delivery.

Pituitary Gland
A gland at the base of the brain that makes hormones that control the functions of other glands of the body.

Placenta
A disc of tissue in close contact with the wall of the uterus. It is connected by two arteries and a vein to embryonic circulation; via the placenta oxygen, foodstuffs, and waste products are exchanged with the mother's circulation. After delivery, the placenta (frequently called the afterbirth) is expelled.

Placenta Previa
A placenta that lies in the lower uterine segment over the cervix and blocking the passage of the fetus through the birth canal.

Preeclampsia
See Toxemia of Pregnancy.

Probability
A measure of predictability with respect to some future event. Probability is the long-run expectation of the relative frequency with which a given event will occur.

Progesterone
A hormone produced by the body to prepare the uterus for the reception and development of the fertilized ovum.

Prolactin

One of the hormones of the anterior pituitary gland that stimulates and sustains lactation in the postpartum period.

Prospective Research

Research that involves gathering information as it becomes available. The obtained facts are used to determine whether any of the information is predictive of particular behaviors or complications.

Retrospective Research

Research that looks backward to what has been experienced in the past. It may rely on an individual's memory or on hospital records.

Risk Factor

The likelihood, or probability, based on available studies and/or statistics that a particular stimulus (e.g., smoking) will cause a particular event (e.g., reduced birth weight).

Sidestream Smoke

Smoke that leaves the lit end of the cigarette between puffs.

Teratogen

A substance that has the capacity to alter normal intrauterine development and so to cause malformations.

Term

The time when a pregnant woman might expect her baby to be born—usually 280 days after the first day of the last menstrual period.

Thalidomide

A sedative drug used in the 1950s and thought at the time to be perfectly safe. Unfortunately, its side effect—severe limb malformations of the unborn child—was not recognized until several thousand babies were affected.

Tolerance

A state of progressively decreasing responsiveness to a drug. As a result more of the drug is needed to get the effect initially felt.

Toxemia of Pregnancy

A condition in which blood pressure rises, fluid is retained in body tissues, making them appear puffy, and sometimes the kidneys' functions are altered.

Trimester

A period of three months into which a pregnancy is divided. Thus, each pregnancy is divided into three trimesters. The first trimester, for example, spans the first three months of pregnancy.

Umbilical Cord

A cord between the placenta and the abdominal region of the fetus. It contains two arteries (carrying blood from the baby to the placenta) and one vein (transporting oxygen-carrying blood from the placenta to the baby).

Uterus or Womb

The hollow organ, suspended in the cavity of the pelvis, in which the fetus grows.

Vitamin C (or Ascorbic Acid)

A vitamin found in fresh fruits and vegetables that is easily destroyed by cooking. Deficiency for a length of time leads to muscular weakness, inflammation of gums, and damage to joints. This substance is also important in the growth of cells. In adults the daily requirement is approximately ten milligrams. During pregnancy an increase of five milligrams is recommended.

Vitamins

A group of substances that exist in small quantities in natural foods and are essential for growth and development.

Villi (Placental)

Tissues that project from the fetal side of the placenta and that are bathed in the mother's blood in the uterus. The transfer of food and oxygen between the mother and the fetus takes place through the walls of the villi.

Withdrawal Symptom

A physiological and behavioral reaction, sometimes severe, that takes place when drug use is abruptly terminated.

Womb

See Uterus.

Zygote

A cell, resulting from the union of a male sperm and a female egg, that divides to become the fertilized ovum.

Suggested Readings
for Each Chapter

Introduction

W. B. Beveridge. *The Art of Scientific Investigation.* New York: Random House, 1957.

This is a nontechnical description of some elements of scientific inquiry. The role of intuition, reason, and strategy and the conduct of experimental work are discussed.

F. Kerlinger. *Foundations of Behavioral Research.* New York: Holt, Rinehart & Winston, 1964.

A very thorough coverage of many aspects of research in the social sciences and the fallacies to be avoided.

R. Kirk. *Statistical Issues: A Reader for the Behavioral Sciences.* Monterey: Brooks-Cole, 1972.

An interesting collection of articles that delve into the logical bases and assumptions of statistics. Incorrect applications are also discussed.

J. Tanur and F. Mostellar (eds.). *Statistics: A Guide to the Unknown.* San Francisco: Holden-Day, 1972.

These nontechnical essays on the use of statistics discuss at a basic level picking subjects, probability, prediction, and decisionmaking.

Chapter 1. Who Are the Smokers?

Health Protection Branch. *Smoking Habits of Canadians, 1965–1974.* Canadian Department of National Health and Welfare, Ottawa: Queen's Printer, 1975.

Health Protection Branch. Smoking Habits of Canadians,

1975. Canadian Department of National Health and Welfare, Ottawa: Queen's Printer, 1976.

Public Health Service. *Adult Use of Tobacco, 1975.* United States Department of Health, Education and Welfare, Washington, D.C.: U.S. Government Printing Office, 1976.

These U.S. and Canadian government publications provide the most complete information about who the smokers were in the years they survey. Numerous details are provided, including a breakdown of smokers by age, sex, employment, education, and region.

P. N. Lee. *Tobacco Consumption in Various Countries.* London Tobacco Research Council. Tobacco Research Council, 1975.

This publication gives a picture of the changing trends in smokers from 1950 to 1975 in a number of countries including the United Kingdom, France, Sweden, Canada, and the United States.

Ontario Department of Health, Perinatal Mortality Study Committee. *Report of the Perinatal Mortality Study in Ten Teaching Hospitals in Ontario.* Toronto: 1967.

This large study, referred to frequently throughout our book, contains an enormous amount of information. The data were collected from births in ten teaching hospitals in Ontario in 1960–1961; over fifty thousand subjects were involved. Further analysis of specific aspects of the data in the study have been subsequently published in several shorter articles, some of which complete the reading list for this chapter.

J. Andrews and J. M. McGarry. "A Community Study of Smoking in Pregnancy." *Journal of Obstetrics and Gynaecology of the British Commonwealth* (1972), vol. no. 79, 12, pp. 1057–1073.

E. B. Hook. "Changes in Tobacco Smoking and Ingestion of Alcohol and Caffeinated Beverages during Early Pregnancy: Are These Consequences, in Part, of Feto-Protective Mechanisms Diminishing Maternal Exposure to Embryotoxins?" In *Birth Defects: Risks and Consequences.* Edited by S. Kelly, E. B. Hook, D. T. Janerich, and I. H. Porter. New York: Academic, 1976. Section IV, 2nd paper.

This chapter contains a discussion of factors that caused

some women to give up or reduce smoking (as well as drinking alcohol and coffee) early in pregnancy.

S. Kullander and B. Kaellen. "A Prospective Study of Smoking and Pregnancy." *Acta Obstetrica et Gynecologica Scandinavica* (1971), vol. 50, 1, pp. 83–94.

These studies, the first a Welsh and the second a Scandinavian report, look at smoking during pregnancy and also at how the habit changes from before to during pregnancy.

M. B. Meyer, J. A. Tonascia, and C. Buck. "The Interrelationship of Maternal Smoking and Increased Perinatal Mortality with Other Risk Factors: Further Analysis of the Ontario Perinatal Mortality Study, 1960–1961." *American Journal of Epidemiology* (1975), vol. 100, no. 6, pp. 443–452.

This publication discusses, among other things, the characteristics of women who smoked during pregnancy.

Chapter 2. Involuntary Smokers

United States Department of Health, Education, and Welfare. "Involuntary Smoking." In *The Health Consequences of Smoking, 1975.* Washington, D.C.: U.S. Government Printing Office, 1975. Chapter 4.

This U.S. government document is a thorough review of the rather limited knowledge in this area. Many interesting figures and examples are given of carbon monoxide concentrations in particular situations.

L. D. Longo. "The Biological Effects of Carbon Monoxide on the Pregnant Woman, Fetus, and Newborn Infant." *American Journal of Obstetrics and Gynecology* (1977), vol. 129 (1), pp. 69–103.

This article is the definitive review of the physiological effects and clinical implications of carbon monoxide exposure in the mother-to-be and her baby.

Chapter 3. Constituents of Smoke

Royal College of Physicians of London. "The Chemistry and Pharmacology of Tobacco Smoke." In *Smoking and Health Now.* London: Pitman Medical, 1971. Chapter 3.

United States Department of Health, Education, and Welfare. "Harmful Constituents." In *The Health Consequences of Smoking: A Report of the Surgeon General.* Washington, D.C.: U.S. Government Printing Office, 1972. Chapter 9.

These chapters from British and American government reports provide a general review of the constituents of smoke. They are much less detailed than Schmeltz's *Chemistry of Tobacco and Tobacco Smoke* mentioned below but both chapters give a very complete list of references for each component of smoke so that the interested reader could pursue an individual compound.

Royal College of Physicians of London. *Smoking or Health: The Third Report from the Royal College of Physicians of London.* London: Pitman Medical, 1977.

These readings present evidence for considering cigarette smoking an addiction.

M. A. H. Russell. "Cigarette Smoking: Natural History of a Dependence Disorder." *British Journal of Medical Psychology* (1971), vol. 44, (1) pp. 1–16.

I. Schemltz. *The Chemistry of Tobacco and Tobacco Smoke.* New York: Plenum, 1972.

This is a collection of papers presented at a symposium on the chemical composition of tobacco and new methods to identify constituents. This is a technical book but for the reader with a knowledge of organic chemistry it is quite informative.

Chapter 4. Mother's Weight Gain during Pregnancy

G. Chamberlain. "The Development of the Embryo." In *The Safety of the Unborn Child.* London: Penguin Hammondsworth Medical Services, 1969.

This chapter presents a good general description of the development of the fetus.

D. P. Davies, O. P. Gray, P. C. Ellwood, and M. Abernethy. "Cigarette Smoking in Pregnancy: Association with Maternal Weight Gain and Fetal Growth. *Lancet* (February 1976), vol. 1, pp. 385–387.

D. Rush. "Examination of the Relationship between Birth Weight, Cigarette Smoking during Pregnancy, and Maternal Weight Gain." *Journal of Obstetrics and Gynaecology of the British Commonwealth* (1974), vol. 81, no. 10, pp. 746–752.

The authors of these reports, relying on careful statistics but rather small samples, conclude that maternal smoking affects birth weight primarily through effects upon the mother rather than upon the fetus. They argue that the reduced maternal weight gain they found among smokers has a nutritional foundation.

G. Mau. "Smoking and the Fetus." *Lancet* (May 1976), vol. 1, no. 7966 p. 972.

M. B. Meyer. "How Does Maternal Smoking Affect Birth Weight and Maternal Weight Gain?" *American Journal of Obstetrics and Gynecology* (1978), vol. 131, pp. 888–893.

These authors interpret their data to show that smoking does not affect maternal weight gain but does reduce the birth weight of the newborn.

S. R. Williams. "Nutritional Guidance in Prenatal Care." In *Nutrition in Pregnancy and Lactation.* Edited by B. S. Worthington, J. Vermmersch, and S. R. Williams. St. Louis: Mosby, 1977. Annex II.

This chapter discusses maternal weight gain, what factors contribute to the increased weight, and nutritional needs during pregnancy.

Chapter 5. The Placenta

Boston Children's Medical Center. *Pregnancy, Birth, and the Newborn Baby.* New York: Dell, Delacorte Press, 1972.

C. Lerch and V. Bliss. *Maternity Nursing.* Third edition. St. Louis: Mosby, 1978

These comprehensive guides to pregnancy and childbirth contain, in approximately twenty pages, clear, brief descriptions of the placenta—its function, structure, and some complications that may arise.

P. Lehtovirta and M. Forss. "The Acute Effect of Smoking on Intervillous Blood Flow of the Placenta." *British Journal of*

Obstetrics and Gynaecology (1978), vol. 85, no. 10, pp. 729–731.

R. L. Naeye. "Effects of Maternal Cigarette Smoking on the Fetus and Placenta." *British Journal of Obstetrics and Gynaecology* (1978), vol. 85, no. 10, pp. 732–737.

These are two of the most recent studies that have looked at smoking, the placenta, and blood flow.

Chapter 6. Complications during Pregnancy

J. Andrews and J. M. McGarry. "A Community Study of Smoking in Pregnancy." *Journal of Obstetrics and Gynaecology of the British Commonwealth* (1972), vol. 79, no. 12, pp. 1057–1073.

R. Butler, H. Goldstein, and E. M. Moss. "Cigarette Smoking in Pregnancy: Its Influence on Birth Weight and Perinatal Mortality. *British Medical Journal* (1972), vol. 2, no. 4, pp. 127–130.

S. Kullander and B. Kaellen. "A Prospective Study of Smoking and Pregnancy." *Acta Obstetrica et Gynecologica Scandinavica* (1971), vol. 50, no. 1, pp. 83–94.

M. B. Meyer, J. A. Tonascia, and C. Buck. "The Interrelationship of Maternal Smoking and Increased Perinatal Mortality with Other Risk Factors: Further Analysis of the Ontario Perinatal Mortality Study, 1960–1961." *American Journal of Epidemiology* (1975), vol. 100, no. 6, pp. 443–452.

R. L. Naeye. "Relationship of Cigarette Smoking to Congenital Anomalies and Perinatal Death." *American Journal of Pathology* (1978), vol. 90, no. 2, pp. 289–293.

These five studies are representative investigations, based on American, Canadian, British, Welsh, and Scandinavian data, of the interaction of smoking and other risk factors during pregnancy. Approximately 140,000 births were investigated by these authors.

Chapter 7. Fetal Growth, Birth Weight, and Prematurity

R. J. Hickey, R. C. Clelland, and E. J. Bowers. "Maternal Smoking, Birth Weight, Infant Death, and the Self-selection

Problem." *American Journal of Obstetrics and Gynecology* (1978), vol. 131, no. 7, pp. 805–811.

In this article the argument is put forth that low birth weight is more related to the smoker than to smoking.

H. V. Meredith. "Relation between Tobacco Smoking of Pregnant Women and Body Size of Their Progeny: A Compilation and Synthesis of Published Studies." *Human Biology* (1975), vol. 47, no. 4, pp. 451–472.

This article lists in tables the results of over fifty studies that compared the birth weights of infants born to smokers and nonsmokers. The author also presents a comparison of black and white mothers who smoke and who do not.

R. L. Naeye. "Effects of Maternal Cigarette Smoking on the Fetus and Placenta." *British Journal of Obstetrics and Gynaecology* (1978), vol. 85, no. 10, pp. 732–737.

A very convincing, large study linking smoking and low birth weight in which mothers who smoked during one pregnancy but not during another had smaller babies after the pregnancy in which they had smoked.

United States Department of Health, Education, and Welfare. "Pregnancy and Infant Health." In *Smoking and Health.* Washington, D.C.: U.S. Government Printing Office, 1979. Chapter 8.

This publication summarizes most of the recent scientific literature on birth weight and smoking. It also has a very thorough list of references for this area.

See also Andrews and McGarry, "A Community Study," and Kullander and Kaellen, "A Prospective Study" (listed in full for Chapter 1); Meyer, "How Does Maternal Smoking Affect Birth Weight" (listed in full for Chapter 4); and Butler, Goldstein, and Moss, "Cigarette Smoking in Pregnancy" (listed in full for Chapter 6).

Chapter 8. The Newborn

T. B. Brazelton. "Why Your New Baby Behaves That Way." *Redbook* (1978), pp. 39–42.

A description of and the rationale for the Brazelton

Neonatal Assessment Scale presented by the physician who originated the testing procedure.

G. Gennser, K. Marsal, and B. Brantmark. "Maternal Smoking and Fetal Breathing Movements." *American Journal of Obstetrics and Gynecology* (1975), vol. 123, no. 8, pp. 861–867.

This study demonstrated a relationship between the smoking of cigarettes by the pregnant woman and the breathing movements of her unborn baby.

The Longo article, "The Biological Effects of Carbon Monoxide" (listed in full for Chapter 2) describes some of the consequences in the newborn of fetal exposure to carbon monoxide.

The suggested readings for Chapter 11 give references that describe symptoms in adults that are associated with giving up smoking.

D. W. Saxton. "The Behaviour of Infants Whose Mothers Smoke in Pregnancy." *Early Human Development* (1978), vol. 2–4, pp. 363–369.

This study, which used the Brazelton scale, found an association between smoking during pregnancy and the hearing of the newborn.

Chapter 9. Breast Milk and Nursing

The first two suggested readings for Chapter 5 contain information about the anatomy of the breasts, the role of hormones in nursing, and the formation, excretion, and nutritional content of breast milk.

The few studies that have looked at the possible interaction between maternal smoking and breastfeeding are outlined in the U.S. government report that is suggested reading for Chapter 7.

Chapter 10. Long-term Effects

N. R. Butler and H. Goldstein. "Smoking in Pregnancy and Subsequent Child Development." *British Medical Journal* (1973), vol. 4, no. 12, pp. 573–575.

H. G. Dunn, A. K. McBurney, S. Ingram, and C. M. Hunter. "Maternal Cigarette Smoking during Pregnancy and the Child's Subsequent Development. (Part 1): Physical Growth to the Age of 6½ Years." *Canadian Journal of Public Health* (1976), vol. 67, no. 6, pp. 499–505.

H. G. Dunn, A. K. McBurney, S. Ingram, and C. M. Hunter. "Maternal Cigarette Smoking during Pregnancy and the Child's Subsequent Development. (Part 2): Neurological and Intellectual Maturation to the Age of 6½ Years." *Canadian Journal of Public Health* (1977), vol. 68, no. 1, pp. 43–49.

J. B. Hardy and E. D. Mellits. "Does Maternal Smoking during Pregnancy Have a Long-term Effect on the Child?" *Lancet* (1972), vol. 2, pp. 1332–1336.

These studies looked at physical and intellectual functioning in children ranging in age from four to eleven whose mothers had smoked during pregnancy.

R. Denson, J. L. Nanson, and M. A. McWatters. "Hyperkinesis and Maternal Smoking." *Canadian Psychiatric Association Journal* (1975), vol. 20, no. 3, pp. 183–187.

This study found that mothers of hyperactive children are more likely to have been heavy smokers when pregnant than are mothers of normal children.

J. G. Wilson. *Environment and Birth Defects.* New York: Academic, 1973.

The first two chapters of this book provide an overview of the study of adverse effects of environmental factors on the fetus (teratogenesis) and also describe the changing susceptibility during various developmental stages and the mechanisms involved.

Chapter 11. Conclusions and Alternatives

E. Garfield. "Nicotine Addiction Is a Major Medical Problem: Why So Much Government Inertia?" *Current Contents* (July 30, 1979), no. 31, pp. 5–13.

This overview by a self-confessed antismoker presents a number of controversial points of view on the addictive properties of nicotine and the success and failure of various approaches used to stop smoking.

J. H. Jaffe and M. E. Jarvik. "Tobacco Use and Tobacco Use Disorder." In *Psychopharmacology: A Generation of Progress.* Edited by M. A. Lipton, DiMascio, and K. F. Killam. New York: Raven, 1978.

This thorough review outlines the psychological, behavioral, and physiological consequences of reducing or stopping smoking. It also discusses different treatments to assist people in stopping their use of tobacco.

Index

143

Weight *(cont.)*
  of newborn, 4, 36, 60–73, 104–106
Weight gain of mothers
  and pregnancy, 4, 33–39, 69–70
  and smoking, 37, 68, 118–119, 120–121

Withdrawal symptoms
  in adults, viii, 27–28, 84–85, 113–114, 117–120
  in newborns, 28, 85–86
Women's liberation, 9